DADDY'S GIRL

In that first moment, the moment of March 1982, when Daddy punished me for the first time, and I was so pleasured and aroused and grateful and mortified and confused, my naughty self danced as a shadow around the room, liberated. I didn't discuss these fleeting notions at this moment, of course I did not. They ebbed away as smoothly as they had arrived and left me in a present full of desperate sexual need.

Daddy got up and stood behind me. He was wearing soft black wool trousers cut narrowly at the waist and wide at the leg – a shape developed in the 1930s and made fashionable by David Bowie. Daddy always looked wonderful. He was very tall and very lean, with a slim waist, long legs, narrow shoulders, but strong arms, as I had discovered. His dick was big. I would not have been interested if it had not been. He stood behind me, and I felt him tall. He stroked my neck, then his fingers went down my back and gently fondled my poor smacked buttocks.

'Ah, Stella,' he whispered, 'my darling. Your Daddy is here and he loves you.'

Overwhelmed I swung around and kissed him as I had never kissed anyone before, with love and passion and long long minutes where there is only the present and nobody can part.

DADDY'S GIRL

Stella Back

First published in 2007 by
Virgin Books
Thames Wharf Studios
Rainville Rd
London W6 9HA

A catalogue record of this book is available from
the British Library

ISBN 978 0 7535 1280 7

The paper used in this book is a natural, recyclable product
made from wood grown in sustainable forests.
The manufacturing process conforms to the regulations of the
country of origin.

Typeset by TW Typesetting, Plymouth, Devon

Printed in the UK by CPI Bookmarque, Croydon, CR0 4TD

To Tim Woodward,
who has done much to enlighten the world.

Dear All,

Having written two erotic novels, I have now
been asked to describe the sexual experiences on
which they were based. This book is based on
my own story and describes an older man with
whom I was involved from 1982–9. I loved him
very much. The details are drawn from the
diaries that I have written all my life, but all
names have been changed, as have some
locations, in order to provide privacy for the
participants.

Love Stella
London 2007
thestellablack@yahoo.co.uk

1. 1982

He had a lot of imagination and his imagination was entirely involved in the creation of sexual scenery and sensual drama. He had the time. His working hours, such as they were, involved the maintenance of his possessions and the movement of his money. He had inherited it when he was 28 and now it involved accounts in the Cayman Islands and a fax machine and late-night telephone calls. He spent hours reading the *Financial Times* and staring at share prices. I did not know how rich he was, but his house in Cheyne Walk was like the Sir John Soane's Museum without the curators. You couldn't move for occasional tables and polished walnut escritoires with inlaid mother of pearl and provenance.

People would stare when he told me off, not realising that I loved it, loved being instructed.

'Come here!'

'No.'

He would smack me with the flat of his hand, on my buttocks, on my thighs, front and back, on and on, until he smelled and felt and heard my genuine supplication. I was always wet and weeping and desperate for him.

Ah me. There's nothing like romance.

I had not been aware that it was possible to realise the images of the inner life. I had often hoped it was possible, but where to find the ally? Where to find the man with the necessary courage, mastery, imagination, generosity and wisdom? Where to find the unembarrassed uncontained person willing to abandon himself to giving pleasure to a naughty girl?

Here he was.

Daddy appeared as if he had been invoked. I met him at a party in a big house in London. There was champagne, an old pop star and a room full of red faces and black dinner jackets.

I am small. Not as small as the Queen, but around five foot five – up to seven with the shoes. I am narrow – boyish I suppose it could be said – and would be more so if it wasn't for breasts that are slightly, but not absurdly, bigger than they should be. And I am dark: dark fringe, dark lashes, dark brow, dark soul. So there I was, in green moiré, cinched-in waist, entertaining décolleté, thin black spikes, seamed stockings.

After twenty minutes of being breathed on by bores, I went to explore the residence, which was one of those places with an indoor pool, Ionic pillars and several original Chagalls. I guess the host must have been one of those rare individuals possessed of both money and taste.

On the third floor I found a bathroom the size of an apartment with two marble sinks, mirrors and a free-standing bath, around which there was an impressive parade of Floris. So I poured in geranium. Who wouldn't? Well. The Bishop of Carlisle might not, but everyone else would. I whooshed it up in the surge from the (real) Victorian taps.

Off came the dress, a green pool on the bath mat; out came a natural sponge the size of my head.

I was relaxing, supine, in delicious hot waves of geranium scent, when he walked in. I was, of course, completely naked, though my modesty, such as it is, was protected to an extent by the high white walls of the Victorian bath.

He didn't say sorry. He hardly looked at me. At first I thought he had not noticed me, which was a unique feeling for me. I am always noticed. I ensure that it is so.

He simply padded across the soft white carpet, pulled out his dick and went to the loo. I did not provide the gratification of staring at either him or it. Then he sat on the edge of the bath and looked at me through the steam.

I didn't say anything but looked him straight in the eye and soaped myself, particularly my breasts, which weren't particularly dirty in the usual sense of the word. Then, still looking at him, I pushed my hand between my legs and rubbed myself. He smiled but he was still silent.

I stood up and rinsed myself with the shower, ensuring that he was allowed the full advantage of a rear view that, with thoughtful presentation, could cause a bus to crash into the back of a police car.

I have a perfect bum. I just do. I can't help it. People are always talking about it and I show it to anyone who asks. There weren't any thongs in the 1980s but if there had been I would have worn them.

I lay back into the water, legs spread, toes on the edges, little crimson nails winking at him, little crimson lips slightly parted to reveal my clit.

He took his time, but we both knew it was up to him to lead. The water nearly went cold. I'm not a patient person and neither do I sit in cold water for any man. At last he stood up and gathered a vast white towel from the silver rails.

'Come to Daddy,' he said. 'It's time for bed.'

I was home.

I remember the first time.

I was 23 but you might not have known it to see me lying on my stomach on the bed in his house, polka-dot cotton knickers and matching socks, reading the *Beano* and eating sweets.

I am Lolita, I thought. But can you be a Lolita and conscious of it? Can you be a Lolita on purpose? Perhaps a woman cannot be a Lolita unless a man decrees that it is so, in the same way that a tree may not make a noise if there is nobody to hear it? The girl is made by the beholder, she cannot be her own creation. Can a nymph think? Can a nymph be a nympho?

Perhaps you think my aspirations were a little distorted – that I was a grown woman and should have been aiming higher than lying around in some rich father-figure's house being pleased with myself. Or perhaps you wish you were me, unless you wish you were Daddy! My hero. Permanently hard and in control and getting everything he wanted.

As I turned the coloured pages of the *Beano*, some chocolate stained the counterpane of his bed and he was furious. 'For God's sake, Stella,' he said. 'It's eighteenth-century silk. You can't dry-clean it, it will destroy it.'

'Well, it's very stupid to have it on the bed then,' I responded, popping another sweet into my mouth. 'Give it to the V&A or something.'

I turned the page to Dennis the Menace and Gnasher.

He didn't say anything, simply took the *Beano* off the bed and placed it on the bedside table. Then he took the sweets and put them on top of it. He walked over to the dressing table where, amongst a line of antique clothes brushes, there was a silver-backed hairbrush that had once belonged to an aged aunt.

He grabbed me, spread me over his knee and ripped down my knickers so that my bare buttocks were presented to him. Then he beat me with all the strength of his right arm.

I was overwhelmed by complete and utter and abject mortification. I went somewhere very young and very hidden and very difficult to articulate. I didn't know where I was, exactly. Physically, I was face down, my buttocks were bare and exposed, my cunt and arsehole were his for the taking.

His strength was overwhelming and I had to surrender to my first ever sexual punishment. He spanked me on the buttocks, he spanked me on the top of the thighs. Then, waiting a minute to survey the crimson marks, he spanked me again, hard, on top of those marks.

I tried to escape, wriggling and complaining, then shouting and threatening. But he merely placed his leg between my thighs so that I couldn't move.

The sound rang out as slaps into the room. The stings became harder and my flesh hotter. I yelped. Then the erotic flush turned into red pain. He slapped my thighs and then returned to my arse, again and again, for about twenty minutes until the arousal and discomfort melded and I eased into the true transcendence of total submission.

He went all the way, spanking me, fingering me, spanking me again. I burst into loud childish sobs. Overcome by humiliation and hot pain and an overpowering need to feel him inside me, I wept. 'I'm sorry. I'm sorry. I won't do it again.'

'No you won't. Stand up with your back towards me.'

I struggled to my feet, dishevelled and tearful. My pants had been pushed down to my knees. I stepped out of them with as much dignity as I could muster. All sensation throbbed to the lower half of my body, buttocks blazing, cunt pulsing. Desperate. I put my hands into my wet pussy. My fingers disappeared into the flesh. I was open. Very open. I had never been so consciously vulnerable in my life. And now I had to enter a place where I trusted this man completely. Trusted him not to actually abuse me. Trusted him not to hurt me.

It was a fine line. How would he or I know when to stop? How far would we go now we had started? Would there be blood, battle scars? Filthy humiliation? Danger? I could already feel the drama of the compulsion to explore.

'Take your hand away from your pussy, Stella.' His voice was not raised; it was firm, sure of being obeyed, but the timbre was one of a man providing unarguable facts rather than a stock character delivering orders. 'You should know now that you will never put your hands near yourself unless I have told you that you may. Do you understand me?'

'Yes,' I said.

I took my hand away from myself.

He sat on the edge of the bed and looked at my back and arse, as if studying a picture in an empty gallery.

I looked good naked, I knew that. My bottom was firm and round and annoying; as were my tits, which had been admired since their welcome (though late) arrival around my eighteenth birthday. I had been a boy until that point, really. I didn't mind. I looked good in boy clothes and they were easier to dance in. I attracted ladyboys and I didn't mind that either since they were always more fun.

I was a beautiful gift for Daddy; a work of art. Comforted by proud vanity I was of the annals of Ingres and Rodin; perfect and white. This was not porno. I was not a reader's wife. I did not think of myself as part of the lewd exhibitions of pervery – the schoolgirls and nurses – but more the sublime exhibition of martyred beauty. But now I was a young girl, naked and red, red in the face and red on the backside. I was being admired by a man silenced by the bruised beauty that he had created.

Daddy liked to look, he liked to watch me walk towards him, naked, in the candlelight, moving towards him slowly down the dark corridor. Then he would send me back again and tell me to walk towards him more slowly, more erect, and then, when I arrived there if front of him, I had to perform some small act of submission. Bob a curtsy, perhaps, or kneel down in front of him so that he could help me up.

He never asked me to kiss his shoes, and I wouldn't have wanted to. We weren't in a period drama, after all; sexualising second-rate screenplays would be too panto for me. Too like making out with Farcy Darcy. I did not kiss the Daddy's shoes, nice though they were, always brogues from Church's. I did occasionally polish them when really pushed, really wanting to please him, or genuinely contrite about a misdemeanour.

Sometimes when Daddy called, I went towards him in a long nightdress with pie-crust frill, clean from the bath, warm and wet, and this was the goodnight kiss. He would take me by the hand, lead me into the bedroom, tuck me up, turn out the light, leave a light on in the corridor and leave to perform some adult duty to which I was not party. Neither did I wish to be. Daddy's activities were dull. He played bridge, for a start. He went to those parties where you have to stand up for an hour and a half.

In that first moment, the moment of March 1982, when Daddy punished me for the first time, and I was so pleasured and aroused and grateful and mortified and confused, my naughty self danced as a shadow around the room, liberated. I didn't discuss these fleeting notions at this moment, of course I did not. They ebbed away as smoothly as they had arrived and left me in a present full of desperate sexual need.

Daddy got up and stood behind me. He was wearing soft black wool trousers cut narrowly at the waist and wide at the leg – a shape developed in the 1930s and made fashionable by David Bowie. Daddy always looked wonderful. He was very tall and very lean, with a slim waist, long legs, narrow shoulders, but strong arms, as I had discovered. His dick was big. I would not have been interested if it had not been. He stood behind me, and I felt him tall. He stroked my neck, then his fingers went down my back and gently fondled my poor smacked buttocks.

'Ah, Stella,' he whispered, 'my darling. Your Daddy is here and he loves you.'

Overwhelmed I swung around and kissed him as I had never kissed anyone before, with love and passion and long long minutes where there is only the present and nobody can part.

He kissed back, withdrew and pushed me gently down onto the bed so I was face up and looking into his face, eye to eye. He lifted up my legs and pushed them over my head. Then he slid a lubed finger into my back passage. 'Play with yourself, Stella. I want you to relax.'

So I rubbed myself and brought myself slowly to the edge of orgasm, as he slid his awful finger in and out of my anal passage, feeling for the sensitivity, stretching to allow himself in, encouraging me to do as I was told.

I obeyed.

He kissed me on the lips.

'Kneel on the floor, with your arse towards me, and your face on the edge of the bed.'

He left the room and I knelt alone for a minute or two. My red cheeks presented. My cunt wet. My arse ready for him. My flushed cheeks on the antique silk. And slowly, his dick wrapped in rubber, he eased himself into me. Very gently. In and further in. I was kneeling and snivelling and moaning but allowing him through.

Then there was only me and him and his dick and my anus. I was dominated and young and very naughty. He was a bad man and he was in a rude place. But I liked it. It was comforting and it pleased him and so I liked it more.

Somewhere there were our smells and the smell of chocolate. He started to thrust harder, letting himself go.

He hugged me. I wept again, overwhelmed by emotion and new sensation and unfamiliar stimuli.

I had a bust and legs and pussy all ready to go but the emotional core of a girl who was searching for something big and male and perfect. Deep down there were parts of me of which I could only ever be vaguely aware, but with which he became involved, and which could only be touched thorough erotic emotional play and penetrative sex.

Daddy's dominance touched forgotten memories and brought them to the surface. He was generous and powerful and knew how to use his dick to find things out about women beyond their technical ability to have an orgasm. He was perfect because he wasn't informed by sex guides or expectations or the absurd mission of finding the clitoris as if it were hidden in some place in Borneo that had only just been discovered. He didn't fall in with that; I don't think he had been informed by the media. I think he had been informed by himself and by the women of his life, of whom there had been many. He had a talent for discovering intimate truths.

My childhood, if it could be called that, was an odd one. The early years were in a house full of cupboards containing monsters that were scaly and furry and whispering and scary. The mother was not there. A male person put me to bed. My father. He was nice and he loved me and then he went and didn't come back.

The father and the mother went, but the mother had already gone before the father and before I could remember her, so her disappearance was never of significance. I was a baby. It didn't matter. She had a tumour, actually, so that was that. The father though came and went in my earliest memories. Then he went out of them and never returned. I expect I was about six when he died, so it would have probably been around 1965.

I can't remember how long it was before I realised that he was not coming back. I used to sit on the edge of my bed, night after night, for quite a long time, staring at the wallpaper, with its design of sweet peas. Legs swinging, staring into space, then palpitating with the horrors of the invisible. Flower pots full of indescribable evil. Noises that heralded the disasters caused by the discarnate. Dolls were alive.

Cybermen and Daleks had never been frightening when he was around but now they were appalling and the voices heard long after the television was turned off.

I became (briefly) religious because I was alone and scared and, looking back, I was right to be. I prayed to God, who, according to somebody at school, was also called 'The Father', so I thought they were one and the same; he who checked the cupboards for mutants and laughed in the face of Dalek extermination, and He who forgave us our trespasses. They were the same person. But neither He nor he nor anyone looked after me and I faced the world alone. Rather muddled. Muddled about where and who I was. Muddled about men and power. I did not understand how God was my Father and he lived in Heaven, but had somehow managed to write the Bible and also be a distant shadow of a frustrating memory.

Nobody explained anything, so I worked it all out for myself. I worked it all out wrong, I expect, except there was nobody to tell me what was right and wrong.

I couldn't ask my grandmother, really, as her drinking disallowed discourse. She spoke in surreal non sequiturs and occasionally walked into the laundry cupboard thinking it was the front door. She once left the house for a month, without a suitcase, and then returned saying she had been in Monaco playing shimmy.

Everyone was horrified but I adored her. Her hats were fantastic and she drove her Austin Healey at 60 mph round Shaftesbury. But she never told me anything.

So my grandmother would lie face down on the floor in the hall, occasionally laughing, sometimes sobbing, often unconscious, while my father remained a mystery that was deep in the memory cells of the parasympathetic system where there were old stories of omnipotent robots and girly princes whose mission it was to destroy all or save me, depending on the mood. I assumed the mood was mine rather than theirs, but I was so involved with them all it was difficult to know what was what half the time. I was hardly seven after all; I still thought that real nuns stood behind the cinema screen to sing the songs in *The Sound of Music*.

I knew that, somewhere out there, there was a male person destined to protect me from everything that was frightening. There was a deep longing for a man who was easy to admire and before whom all enemies fell. A man whose style reflected self-confidence and insouciance and a mighty intelligence gathered from many planets over centuries of time travel.

I was missing something. I didn't know what it was, but the symbols of the void, the grief, the atrophy, whatever it was, or is, arrived in the form of spectacular figments whose guises were many and varied, but always controlled and in control.

'Why do we like this?' I once asked him, after a particularly strict session. He had caned me for the first time. It was agony but I was enjoying the afterburn.

We were both lying face down, naked, on his bed in the London house. There were tears on my thoroughly disgruntled face, my arse was up in the air, six livid weals being cooled by the exposure. His hand was stroking me, from my neck, to my back, to the protuberances that he had made.

It was after lunch. Sunday. Winter was settling in outside. We had been seeing each other for over a year.

'Not so much *this* as *you*,' he replied. 'I like you. Love you actually. I think you're wonderful. I don't know why I'm wired to enjoy control, but I do, and I like the effect that it has on you. There is something about you that is vulnerable and needs to be defended, so I think that I must do that, that I must protect you from the dangerous side of your proclivities.

'You enjoy a certain amount of physical pain, but you need someone to watch out for the dangers of this. This form of protection makes me hard – primal, I guess. I expect I am protecting the receptacle of my seed or something.

'And I love that I am old and you are young. I like it when you are bad and confused and asking for it.

'There have been other women, of course there has, but in general they pretended and it wasn't authentic. They played because they were more interested in my money than they were in me. It was never very interesting. I mean, I came and it was nice and all that, but our minds were never engaged. This didn't matter so much when I was younger, but now it does. As one grows older one becomes more bored. I like to come as much as any other man, but I prefer it if there is a dimension that works not only for my mind and body, but for the other person's mind and body as well.

'If this requires unconventional foreplay, so be it. I have never believed that the bedroom should have boundaries. It should be private and safe for the two adults in it. And if more women understood this, less men would go to go prostitutes. If more men understood it, less women would give up on their libidos after their second child.

'You are my perfect naughty girl. Our libidos match. Both of us want as much sex as the other. And this in itself is unusual, let me tell you. I am fifty. Women go off it. They particularly go off it when they have received what they want in the form of legal rights, medical insurance, carpets and babies. Then the poor chap may as well go and fold up his dick and put it on the shelf alongside the newly washed terry-cotton babygros.'

I was thin and demented and wild and confused and he found me and fed me and fucked me and provided order. I didn't know whether I was Martha or Arthur, swinging from one vanilla fuck to the next, imbibing and snorting and smoking and slurping. We all fixed up because Lou Reed did. I didn't think the party was any good unless somebody had died.

I was lucky to find Daddy. He allowed me to feel.

He appeared at exactly the right moment. He would never have allowed me to take drugs, he hated them, and only drank red wine himself. He never gave me any. He said I was too young to drink. And I wasn't allowed to smoke. If there is one thing you learn at boarding school it is how to smoke. It's the only thing, come to think of it. I didn't smoke in front of him for fear of reprimand and punishment. This was complicated, of course, by the fact that I enjoyed both reprimand and punishment. It didn't always work like that though; he was not predictable. Sometimes he did not react to provocation. While my whole body longed for a hot walloping, he would simply take the cigarette out of my mouth, look bored and ignore me. The worst was when he simply dropped me home after dinner. Sometimes that made me cry. It was hardly fair to alter the rules when this game was complicated enough. To one day kiss and smack and fuck and love as a reward for transgression; on another, walk away from the same transgression and leave the disappointed at home in the dark.

Nowadays, now I am old and fierce, I would not allow it. I would demand some kind of mutually agreed coda. Some explanation. But, then, in 1982, he was the Daddy. At some level I thought he knew best. But I still didn't understand. I didn't understand what was going on when he detached from the age play and refused affection. Withheld, as they call it nowadays. I don't know if he did it on purpose or not.

My only defence was to disappear. If he withheld, I withdrew. Gratifyingly this made him furious. There would be a showdown full of drama and need and make-up sex and a good punishment. Our love was always affirmed.

He'd call me on the phone. 'Where have you been? I've been ringing for over a week.'

'Here and there.'

I remember him once telling me, 'Jimmy's coming round in the car in ten minutes. You had better be ready. Wear the white dress I gave you with the white boots and the grey coat, and don't you dare wear pants.'

So I would shower off whatever club or country I had been in, put the hair up in a tousled arrangement which I knew he appreciated, slap on red lipstick and eyeliner, smudge it all, spray over an obscure musk scent I had found on 4th Street in New York and often slip into a little white shift, very short, with white boots – kind of Jackie O in sixth form.

At times like these, when I was the returning miscreant – dark fringe, red lipstick, eyeliner, passport in handbag, being Jane Fonda in *Klute* – when I arrived at his place, Daddy would not greet me in the hall. Jimmy's wife Susan, the housekeeper, would take my coat over her arm, show me into the main drawing room and close the door after me. A fire would be flaring, the yellow and orange flames refracting from the crystal decanters on the drinks tray. The walls were covered in portraits of men in wigs and women in crinolines; there were also cavalier spaniels and stags and bowls of fruit. They would all look down at me, staringly.

So on these evenings when punishment and love and experimentation were in the air, when I had been collected by Jimmy and driven to Daddy's house, I flounced around in the grand drawing room, watched by the oil paintings of tight-lipped women, gun dogs and Georgian fatsos.

The curtains, long and heavy in gold and crimson, would be drawn and it would be quite dark. Daddy would not come for ages. It could be as much as half an hour! I was ready for that, ready for the waiting. I loved to wait. So much could happen in that infernal half an hour, waiting for the authority to arrive and put one right, to whip out the demons, release the internal pain, to cause a crying and a sobbing and fear and loathing and love.

On one particular evening, on a Jackie O/Jane Fonda night, I remember how the minutes ticked by, signified by an eighteenth-century carriage clock on the mantelpiece. I was excited. A tiny clawing started deep in my pelvis, travelled ineluctably towards the internal flesh of my vagina, and pulsed around my lips and clit. I looked forward to his arrival in this room, as I prophesied the pain and pleasure that I was lucky enough to be about to receive from a man who understood me.

My head though, my head was way out of synch. My head wanted to escape the inevitable, get the fucking without the pain! My thoughts were of recalcitrance but immersed in the delicious knowledge that he would win. He was bigger, he was stronger, he was in possession of a huge dick, and I wanted it.

He found me in a state of conscious disarray, dress hitched up my thighs to the edge of my knickers, lounging on the sofa, boots on, fingers inside myself. This was guaranteed to infuriate him, both because the sofa was covered with new upholstery, and he wouldn't want my juices all over it, and because he did not like me to play with myself without permission. He liked watching, he liked to have full control over my orgasm, and usually did.

He appeared, like an eighteenth-century illusionist, a dark figure in the half light.

And on this occasion I hadn't seen him for two weeks. He did not greet me or smile. 'Stand up!'

Stand up for what? I thought. Women's rights? But I didn't dare say this. Daddy didn't do jokes when he was displeased. And he was always telling me that I should stand up when he walked into the room. It was a respect he felt he deserved.

I stayed where I was, staring at him with a mocking smile on my face and a glint in my eye. My heart was beating and I was extremely nervous, but had no intention of showing it.

He pulled me up, tugging me roughly by my arms, and, with one movement, bent me over so that my hands were on the edge of the seat of an armchair. I had hardly got my bearings when the white dress was over my head, and my arse and thighs and puss were his.

He pulled out his hard dick and took me from the back. Just in. No words. No foreplay. A hard silent fuck. And his orgasm was the priority. Protocol was not the order of this scene. My pleasure was not considered – though, of course, we both knew I liked this. I liked him fucking me and coming when he wanted to. And I knew in these moments that I had misbehaved and needed to redeem myself.

He pumped himself into me, came, shuddered, withdrew. I was still folded over the armchair, buttocks in the air, cunt wet, come down my leg, silent. He pulled the shift down, unzipped it, and peeled it from my body. I stepped out of it. I was naked now, except for the soft white leather boots which had been made for me and fitted my calves like opera gloves. They were beautifully pointed and had stiletto heels and they stayed on. My legs were bare. My arse white because I hadn't seen him for two weeks. My puss was neat, black and short but not shaved.

Still silent he pushed me down on all fours on the white rug in front of the fire.

'You wait there and don't move. And don't touch yourself.'

'But I need . . .'

He sighed. 'Don't move. You're a naughty girl.'

I was beginning to want to go to the loo and wondered if I dared to go then and there, feel the warmth down my legs, the childish lack of control, the mess on the rug. He would be incandescent. I decided it wasn't worth it.

My cunt was throbbing and my head was swimming and I hadn't come. But there was an enormous feeling of safety, being so warm and fucked and aroused by his fire. I trusted him, the fire was comforting, the fabrics were soft, the smell of pot-pourri was sweet and sophisticated. I was in the right place.

He left me there for about fifteen minutes, which was just enough time before the genuine discomfort set in with aches.

I sensed him as he returned to the room but I didn't see what he was carrying until he held it in front of my face –

a thin crop made out of willow. He striped my buttocks, neat, sharp and quick, six times, six livid red streaks, parallel, swollen. 'You will not, I repeat, not go away without telling me where you are going.'

I was silent.

He whipped me. 'Do you understand me?'

'Yes, Daddy.'

'You will ring me everyday and tell me where you are.'

'Yes, Daddy.'

'And you know what will happen to you if you do not?'

'Yes, Daddy.'

Naked, the flesh of my buttocks throbbing, still wearing the white boots, I bent into his lap and sucked him the way he liked me to.

Who was in charge now? Who knows? I was on my knees. He was in my mouth. Near my teeth. I had the power but I was the slave. Explain that and stay fashionable.

At this moment he removed himself – slid away from me, so that I was kneeling in front of him, mouth open, gaping like a goldfish.

'Now go to bed,' he said.

'But, you're hard!'

'Go to bed.'

'I still haven't come. I'll never sleep!'

'Go to bed, Stella. I can't believe you're arguing with me after that whipping. Do you want me to beat you again?'

'No thank you.'

My arse was stinging like hell. I would have weals for a week.

Grumbling, I stomped down the corridor as he followed me, catching up with me at one point and delivering a smart slap on my right buttock to show he was displeased with my attitude.

I sat on the bed and removed my white boots.

'Don't sulk,' he said softly, stroking my hair.

With unusual grace he removed his clothes, came to me, still erect and slid deeply into me. We fucked, vanilla in bed. Missionary. Slow and straight like normal people. Now I did come, long and loud and very gratefully. I often laugh when I come. Laughing has always been very sexy for me, very near the physical release of orgasm, those tiny fleeting seconds of transcendence and joy, the welcome escape from the muttering voices and mundane platitudes of the self. I laughed. He smiled.

'You're my own little girl,' he said. As he kissed me, he released himself into me.

He introduced me to the reality of pleasures that had only existed in some ill-formed and fantastic dreams.

I have never believed in indulging guilt. As an emotion it is ego-based and useless, always referring to the person feeling it rather than the person who has been hurt or needs help. The history of guilt describes a spurious concept manufactured by institutions with the purpose of manipulation and as likely to cause amoral conduct as prohibit it. Shame, a different thing, is more insidious, more inherent to the psyche, much more difficult to deflect because it settles in subtle ways before one has noticed what is happening.

I occasionally wondered if I was relatively weird, or whether everybody wanted a 'Daddy' and I was lucky. I did feel lucky. I felt as if my dreams had come true. When I looked at the catwalks, I saw a lot of little girls selling little girl dresses to richer older women. Women with children and careers. For your consideration – selling pink puffball fairy numbers teamed with stripy tights and clumpy Mary Jane shoes, which will make your legs look like that of a child. Why were toddler clothes being sold to grown women? Why were adolescents advertising them? Twenty years later, they still are.

Freud and Jung, always diverting, occasionally tried to explain women for the benefit of their bearded fraternity. They created the idea of the Electra complex after the psychotic Greek goddess, which I take as a compliment, but I don't think it was meant as one. Freud was good on incest but not much of a friend to the sisters. I'm not teaching women's studies in southern California so luckily I don't have to dwell on that too much.

The beards tried to explain the inverse of the Oedipus complex; that is, though devoting most of their studies to the neuroses that were the apparent result of the mother/son relationship, they managed to acknowledge, in passing, that there were also dynamics between father and daughter. Their theory was that the daughter becomes libidinally attached to her father and imagines that she will become pregnant by him. She then turns herself into her mother in order to be attractive to him. Add to this the notion that the incestuous connection (genetic sexual attraction) has to be repressed and the first explanations about the female psyche were about desire and conflict and fear of punishment and Daddy.

Jung did not think there was anything wrong with this; he didn't think the animus/shadow that demanded punishment was sick, he thought it connected with the psyche and aided both self-realisation and a sense of being alive. I thought he was right. Daddy made me come alive; I had never known anything like it. I was not consciously looking for pain in the car-crash, paper-cut, toe-stubbing, head-banging accident sense. I did, however, like getting high; I enjoyed investigating transcendence and was interested in anything that inspired it, which is why I had occasionally taken drugs. The endorphin high, provoked by pain, is a comfortable space. It is calming and helps one feel close to people. Nowadays they call it the 'sub space' but nowadays all this has become very sophisticated.

Wikipedia currently lists both 'Age Play' and 'Daddy's Girl' as accepted and defined fetishes, out there with leather and foot worship, as if they were common and identifiable indulgences, to be enjoyed in the same way as kissing and fondling. Age Play, is, apparently, 'regressive roleplay'. It can cause concern in some people's minds, but for some it can be, 'a healthy or healing outlet'. For others it is like any fantasy in that it allows an 'exploration of feelings'. The Taken in Hand relationship, extolled on the website of the same name, is attracting attention from those who are undoubtedly confused by the difficult differences between the realities of biological make-up and the expectations of society's ever shifting and often paradoxical expectations.

This has all come a long way since I was gadding about in a short skirt and asking for it. The desire to reconstruct old-fashioned ideas about the structures of male/female domestic power dynamics says something about the stress between what some men and women feel as fundamental needs and the political pressure to repress those needs in order to conform to the greater cause of equality. But I did not know all this when I met Daddy. Looking back, I was investigating surrender. I wanted to let go. I wanted to be seen. I knew, on some level, that I had chosen not to be seen. I was aware, in early years, of the use of conscious invisibility as a survival mechanism – if they can't see you they can't make you do something you don't wish to do. Later I discovered the use of conscious visibility – that is, the mask of performance – and indulged in some cabaret appearances in New York. I played a synthesiser like Duran Duran and danced, fuelled into a frenzy by the substances that were available in the East Village and by the flattery of the queens who were on the rampage.

Everyone dressed up then. Nobody was seen. But everybody was acting out their fantasies, so they were dressing up in order to be seen. I wanted Daddy to see my sexual core, to indulge it and to love me for it. I wanted unconditional regard. And I wanted to be saved.

Excuse me. Who doesn't?

2. 1982–3

I loved going shopping with Daddy. Well, of course I did. Expeditions to toy shops were both memorable and delightful. A special treat. Men had bought me jewellery in the past; they didn't understand the toy thing. I didn't really want jewellery, I always lost it anyway. I wanted love, as we all do, and I was cursed with wisdom. I knew that love was more than a bling thing from Tiffany. I knew it was about time and trust. And sex. My tastes were specific. I drew a line at a soft toy, or 'plush' as I think it is now called. If Daddy had bought me a teddy bear I would have been unnerved and angry. A person with a picture of The Slits Sellotaped to their fridge is not a person with a teddy bear on their bed unless its legs have been removed.

Grown women with soft toys in their bedrooms should be avoided with assiduity. Women who attend fairs full of collectable 'character dolls' are also a sinister species, though their darkness is more interesting. The doll's house is a middle ground, I feel, between the demented atrophy of the Sloane Ranger with a teddy bear on her bed and the void of the motherless woman for whom there is no consolation.

Daddy bought me an expensive doll's house from Christies. He said it was an investment. An investment in what? I wondered. In me? In my childhood? In the surreal tableau that we liked to call our affair? Or was what we were doing an actual relationship? 'It is an antique,' he said. 'It will increase in value.'

Jimmy took the doll's house upstairs. It had lights and wallpaper and everything. The detail was magnificent. There were curtains and bedding and china and baskets full of bread. The façade was Georgian and modelled on a house in Belgravia. It had five bedrooms, a kitchen, a drawing room, a nursery, an attic and seemed to offer a lifestyle that was predominately Victorian.

I took the family's clothes off and put them in a pile in the middle of the upstairs bedroom floor.

I had control of the dolls.

Daddy liked to control me.

The first time Daddy took me to a toy shop – a huge place in outer suburbia – he said, 'One toy only!'

'The thing is, I need quite a lot of things for the doll's house. I need a sink, some corner cabinets and a hatstand. I really want a hat stand . . . and the hats come to think of it, they do them. Then there is the cat and the . . .'

'I told you. One toy only and if you argue with me I will take you back into the car park and put you in the car. Do you understand me?'

I considered lying down in the middle of the corridor marked 'Action Toys' and remaining supine until he bought me exactly what I wanted. I was five foot five, after all, and eight stone. Petite in one sense, but difficult to move in another. Still, even I, immersed in lovely fantasy as I was, recognised that a 23-year-old woman having a tantrum in the middle of a toy shop might cause more problems with the security department than was necessary.

He was a kind Daddy, a good Daddy, a cruel Daddy, a perfect lover and role player, but he would not be able to explain himself to the outside world. The outside world would not understand. He looked like any other distinguished businessman in an expensive dark-blue wool coat. He had a high forehead and dark-grey hair and blue eyes. The grey hair suited him; he looked as if he should have been born with it, though in his youth he had been dark. He said I made him go grey but this wasn't true. He was greying when I met him. His teeth were even and white and showed when he smiled. When he smiled, which wasn't often. When he smiled he lost fifteen years as so many people do – the smile reflected past joy. I could see what he had been like when he was younger. In general, though, he was a serious person and difficult to please. Not that I tried very hard to please him, not in the beginning anyway.

When he took me out to the toy shop, I aroused myself with the thought of how far I could push our limits in a public domain. I, being an exhibitionist, would have performed the full perv scenario, believing, as I did, in the validity of using the body in direct action statements. I had seen Karen Finley stick a yam up herself and I had looked into Annie Sprinkle's vagina. I would have taken great pleasure in getting my bum tanned with the general public looking on. Shock tactics suited me.

My early years were devoid of any evidence of emotional warmth and very few, if any, examples of kindness, which is why, when punk rock came along, hard and furious, I knew it was right. My love affairs were scenes of insolence and indignity, both of which were fashionable in 1977. Angry and disassociated, I was at one with the summer of hate. Relationships weren't doctored as they are now; there were no red-lipped termagants issuing edicts about what women should or should not do with their personal lives. We lived in a free-fall free-for-all and fucked as we pleased. If you wanted to be thrown down the stairs to see how it felt then you arranged it. I wouldn't recommend it actually, the thought of it is more interesting than the actuality.

Punk sex. You weren't supposed to have it. John Lydon had pronounced that it was pointless, which was probably more of a reflection on him than anyone else but he was taken very seriously at the time.

I happened to like bending over the loos at the Hope and Anchor and being shafted from the back by a leather boy with neon-green hair. I liked feeling his bony pelvis grind into my bare arse cheeks, feel his beringed fingers on my tits, hear his pleasure. I guess I have always liked it from the back. It is an advantage sometimes not to see their faces, though this can cause confusion later on when they hail you in some club and you don't know who the fuck they are.

I didn't kiss much. Lipstick was very important and always dark purple and, though it looked great smeared all over the face, I found that kissing was best accomplished with men with whom you are very nearly in love. Paradoxically, I kissed girls more indiscriminately and particularly in public, knowing it was a fail-safe way to attract attention.

I liked defying Daddy, pushing him to his limit, but we could only go so far. I did not actually want to make him miserable or embarrassed. In the face of public disturbance or disorder he would have walked away and left me to the authorities. He sat on boards. There were shareholders. Portfolios. Suits. A scandal would have caused him unnecessary inconvenience and made him look a fool.

The outside world, at this moment, was of no importance. We had our world. We were playing. He was hard and I was wet and it was bliss.

'But!' I gazed, lost in the biggest toy shop in the world. Well. That's what the sign said. It was what the retailer believed. The Biggest Toy Shop in the World. This meant a fantastic kingdom of plastic and wood and primary colours. It meant that dolls owned Ferraris and action figures had underwater equipment and snakelike tongues. There were Froggies and Doggies and Playmobil, all of which could be explored for hours on end. I never became tired of it, though the Daddy sometimes became impatient and would take me by the hand and march me to the till.

'I've spoiled you, Stella,' he would say. 'I've spoiled you, and I've created a bad girl.'

Rules were made to be broken. He made them, I broke them. The rules said I was to be polite in the shop, not ask for things, not whine or sulk.

His favourite aisle was entitled 'Dressing Up for Girls and Boys'. This was a hideous gallery of masks and prosthetics: fanged freaks, dragons, one-eyed zombies and scarred Nazis. There was nothing you couldn't get. Your baby could be a monkey, a duckie or a pumpkin. Your son could be a policeman. The teenager could be a cool ghoul, a night slasher or a high seas rogue.

If he makes me be a Tinkerbell I'll never speak to him again, I thought. But the Skeleton Bride was good, as was Dragon Geisha and Zombie Cheerleader. My spirits rose.

'There are nuns,' I informed him.

'You're not being a nun,' he said. 'It's not *Monty Python*. Just stand there.'

A young man appeared. His face was not his advantage. Indeed, his face could easily have taken its place amongst the Halloween masks. He was wearing a green nylon uniform.

'I'm looking for a witch.'

The assistant didn't say, 'Aren't we all?' as I would have

done, but displayed an expression as wide and dry as the Gobi Desert.

'Over here, sir,' he said in the voice of Shaggy from *Scooby-Doo*.

Daddy stroked the back of my neck and, overpowered by fatherliness and his smell and my compulsion to take him into me, I nearly cried.

'I don't want a bloody witch outfit, I want –'

'Don't be rude,' he said calmly, 'I'm putting you in a black net skirt, thigh-high boots, seamed stockings and shiny shiny PVC pants. We're getting the skirt here – the boots and knickers you'll have to wait for and, I might add, I will be caning and buggering you when you are wearing them.'

I knew I would flip myself over for him, let him push the net over my head and cane me, slashing onto the PVC until my flesh started to sweat inside it and I would grow wet into that pervy plastic fabric.

'I don't want the witch!'

Chewing hard, I blew a pink bubble into his face, stared defiantly at him for more than half a minute and walked off in the opposite direction – past shelves piled high with farm animals, past plush badgers, past mighty Action Men with inmate muscles and criminal leers.

I knew he liked the sight of my disappearing rear. He liked my rear in general, and he wasn't the only one. There was a lot of life in those cheeks and it was showing since my white silk shorts were cut halfway up them.

The shoes – black velvet peep-toes with a bow on the toe – were chunky and slightly too big, like Minnie Mouse. They were the most adorable things you have ever seen, a mixture of pure pervert and adorable innocence that it is very difficult to achieve in a shoe. Daddy loved them. Well. He should do. He had bought them.

So off I tottered, head in the air, away from him and his witches' outfits. I disappeared through aisles full of Mermaids and Monopoly and something the Gremlins had bred. Past a 'Winged Puffball', past a knight fighting a dragon with martial moves, until I was lost in every sense, subsumed by thoughts, surrounded by animatronics. And then, oh bliss to behold – Daleks! I nearly died. There they were, in every shape, size and form. Dalek pens, Dalek lunch boxes, remote-controlled Daleks, Dalek T-shirts, Dalek tins. Annihilate. Exterminate. Destroy. I felt a rush of genuine pleasure. Daleks have always made me feel very very happy.

You might ask, and it would be fair to do so, how the terrifying metal maniacs of *Who* lore infiltrated the psychosexuality. But there is a link between terror and safety and sex, my friends.

'Ladies and gentlemen, please note that we will close in ten minutes. Please make your way to the checkout area.'

I don't know how long I had been there but somehow a trolley had filled up with Daleks. I simply don't know how they got there. By themselves, probably, knowing them. If he doesn't let me have these, I thought, I am going to pay for them myself. I'm not leaving this shop without a Dalek and that is all there is to it.

He was waiting at the till. The witch outfit was in a carrier bag. I knew he was about to blow. It was my pleasure to press the button of that detonator.

'Where have you been? I've told you about wandering off.'

'So?'

'Don't you dare speak to me like that!' He was furious. 'The more I give you the more you take.'

'Is that a compliment?'

He pulled my hands away from the bars of the trolley

where they were gripping so hard my knuckles had turned white. He didn't even look down at the Daleks, of which there were about twenty, and one of whose voice-activated mechanism was chanting in the familiar (and well-loved) tone of threat. 'Exterminate. Exterminate. Destroy.'

Daddy was an enemy of the Daleks. Let's face it, everyone was an enemy of the Daleks. Even some Daleks ended up being enemies of the Daleks. I smiled, more because I was amusing myself than because I was mocking him. He glowered and his eyes flashed dangerously.

'I've had enough of you, Stella.'

'But –'

'No.'

'But I want –'

'No.'

'If you don't let me have a Dalek, I am going to scream and it is very likely that you will be arrested.'

'If you utter another word, I will take down your pants and I will spank you here. On your bare bottom, with your shaved puss showing, and I will not stop until you beg me for mercy and perhaps not even then.'

We faced each other in a sexual stand-off, bluffing, seeing who had the nerve to go the furthest.

Daddy won.

I allowed him to win.

People stared as we exited and I was being told off.

Children looked. They didn't know if I was ten or twelve or twenty.

I never knew where the car was parked but Daddy led me to it, clenching my hand so that it began to hurt.

The shops were closing and it was dark. The car park was empty.

Jimmy was leaning against the door on the driver's side smoking a Benson and Hedges. 'Successful trip, sir?'

Daddy didn't say anything, but merely pulled me around to the bonnet of the sedan, pushed my head over it so that my face was down and my arse was raised towards him.

Jimmy ground his fag out with the sole of his immaculate black shoe and got in the driving seat where he watched through the window.

Daddy pulled my little shorts down my thighs and past my knees to my ankles and the tarmac on the ground. No knicks, bare bottom, long socks, heels. He slapped my right buttock with the full force of his hard hand. There were no preliminaries, no more threats, no easing into it with erotic slaps – he just smacked hard. And then another on the left. I yelped as I took five or six hard ones.

'Ow! Ow! Ow! Ow!'

I didn't have time to assess the situation, to think about Jimmy watching us or the risk of being seen.

The pain seared into my arse and took all thoughts away.

Smack. Smack. Smack.

'What do you say?'

'I'm sorry.'

He reached down and picked up my shorts. I rubbed my red cheeks.

'That really hurt!'

'Good.'

He hugged me and helped me gently into the back of the sedan where I lay with my head on his lap and my buttocks naked. I was hot and red and wet and tearful and it made him very hard.

He stroked my hair and kissed me.

'Suck me now.'

I gently pulled his dick out of his flies and placed the head in my mouth, then tenderly kissed it and licked. He pushed his erection into my face and down my throat and I took it all, but I didn't want it there. I wanted it in me.

I pulled my face from between his legs and said, 'I want you to fuck me.'

'You'll have to wait.'

Then he handed me the biggest Dalek of the range. Radio controlled, twelve inch, flashing lights, automated head movement, poseable gun and arm, blast sound effects and authentic voice mechanisms and illuminated eye. 'You make your daddy very happy.'

We went back to Cheyne Walk for tea. Susan served it on a silver tray in front of the fire. I had hot chocolate and cake. Daddy had Earl Grey.

'You had better make the most of that,' he said, 'because you are going to bed.'

'It's six thirty!'

'You're going to bed.'

'I'm not tired.'

'Don't argue with me, please.' Daddy rang the bell.

Susan appeared at the door. She was in her late fifties, with a kind but impassive face. She had allowed her hair to go grey and, unlike Daddy's, it did her no favours. She always wore cardigans and box-pleat skirts and sensible shoes with tan tights. Her only form of creative expression was her pinnies, which sometimes had amusing motifs stamped on them or were evidence of where she and Jimmy had gone for their holidays. Greece, for instance, or Spain.

I once tried to make Daddy speculate on the nature of Susan's underwear but he told me to be quiet.

'Run a bath please, Susan.'

'Yes, sir.' She closed the door behind her.

'I don't want to go there on my own, there might be ghosts.'

'There won't be ghosts,' he said. 'Go and get in the bath and I will come in a minute.'

'Promise?'

'Yes.'

I stomped down the corridor, left my clothes in a pool on the floor and slipped into the tub, which was long enough to lie down in and deep enough to float in the foamy white bubbles. There was a window in front and two basins, one with Daddy's toothbrush and shaving brush – he used soap, the old-fashioned way. The only light came from a bulb on top of the mirror over the basin.

I relaxed, though my bottom was throbbing and all the nerve endings of my pelvis were alive with need.

Daddy appeared after about five minutes, rolled up his shirtsleeves, knelt down on the floor and scrubbed my face with a wet flannel. Then he washed the rest of me with a soft sponge, paying particular attention to the places he considered to be his.

'Stand up.'

He soaped between my legs and I nearly came.

'Daddy!'

He smiled. 'Now. Out.'

He dried me carefully with a white cotton bath blanket.

I caught sight of myself in the mirror. My face was clear of make-up and I was slightly flushed. My hair was wet and in tails. My bush was bare.

He had laid a nightdress out on his huge blue bed. It was white Viyella with a square yoke, long sleeves and broderie anglaise. It was soft and cottony and the hem swept the floor. I put it on and sat on the edge of the bed while he brushed my hair off my face.

'That hurts!'

'No, it doesn't. Now turn over and let me see your bottom.'

I did as I was told and lay stomach down on the bed. He lifted up the nightie to view the marks that his hands had made in the car park.

'Stay there.'

He rattled around in one of his drawers and returned with a pot, the contents of which he gently rubbed onto the marks, which were beginning to go purple. It was so cool, the cream, cool and comforting. I could feel myself beginning to drip for him.

'Get into bed.' He opened the sheets for me. 'In.'

The sheets smelled clean and ironed. He always had three pillows, expensive and soft. I nestled back, small and young. I put my thumb in my mouth. I was regressing, way way back, into a place that I knew was there, but for which there was no actual memory. I felt a serenity of mind that I had never felt before, not even with the best opiates. I forgot who I was. There was only him. I felt like crying. I just wanted to be his.

He read me a feminist fairy story. It was about a girl who lived in a wood and had to save a prince from a snake, which was wound around his neck. I don't know where he got it from. America perhaps.

'And the girl of the woods said goodbye to the prince and good riddance. She lived happily ever after on her own in her own house that she had paid for.'

'Let's have another one.'

'No. Lights out. Bed.'

'But I haven't come. I'll never sleep. It's still really early. Don't go!'

'Goodnight, darling.' He kissed me on the lips and turned the light out.

I couldn't believe it. I was frantic with sexual desire. 'Leave the light on.'

The light in the corridor shone through a crack in the door. I heard his soft footsteps pad back to the sitting room and I felt bereft.

Aroused, abandoned and upset, I could feel my heart beat. Perhaps I should bring myself off. But no, I didn't want myself. I wanted him and I couldn't understand why he didn't want me.

I left it for fifteen minutes but I couldn't bear it. I got out of bed and padded to the sitting room in my bare feet. He was listening to *Rigoletto* and reading a book under his reading light. The fire was still blazing and his shirtsleeves were still up. I stood at the door for a minute, watching his head bent over his book, under the light, until he felt himself being watched and looked up.

'What are you doing there? I told you to go to bed.'

'I can't sleep.'

'Don't whine.'

I walked over to him, stood in front of him, lifted up the white nightie and rubbed my fanny with my hand. 'I want sex and I want it now.'

I stepped over to the rug in front of the fire, lay down, pulled my nightie up and spread my legs so that he could see my needy lips, the swollen clit and the inside of my thighs.

He sighed. If you please. Sighed.

Then he slowly, oh so slowly, took his leather bookmark and carefully placed it in his novel. He is the only person I have met, either then or since, who actually has a leather bookmark with gold tassles and gold letters. He came over and stood over me as I lay on the floor offering myself to him, demented with need. He looked tall and stern and I didn't know what he was going to do next. He did not look pleased.

'You really are a little animal,' he said. 'I've had puppies with more self-control. I should whip your behind and put you straight back to bed.'

I put my fingers up myself, took them out and licked them. 'Please let me play with myself.'

'Get on all fours, Stella. I want to see that perfect arse.'

The perfect arse was still pink from the punishment it had

received earlier. Two naughty crimson orbs peeked up at him framed by the white frills of the nightie.

He knelt down behind me and pushed my face down into the rug where the wool shag tickled my nose. I heard him undo the zip of his flies and, without speaking, he inserted himself hard into me.

I have always been a size queen – it is the way I'm made, I guess. I have a deep dark cunt and a deep dark void in my soul and both need to be filled. When I first encountered Daddy's lucky attribute I thought it was too big, actually, though I hadn't realised there was such a thing. He went into me and I had to concentrate to relax and accommodate, whereas with most dicks I had to concentrate in order to tighten my pelvic floor to allow them to experience that 'tight pussy' they all go on about. But Daddy was large and because he was large it was easier for me to prostrate myself and to show my appreciation. It was easier for me to genuinely love his dick, because I did.

He thrust into me and I cried out loud.

Pushing me further down, his hand on the back of my neck, he thrust again, deep and hard, using his other hand to manipulate me as he did so, playing me.

I came long and loud and very gratefully.

'You're a naughty girl,' he said and, as he kissed me on the back of the neck, he released himself into me while my internal muscles were still pulsing.

He lay on top of me by the fire. He smelled like a man and I felt his weight on me and I never ever wanted to leave that place – the odd place of being crushed by a man. A man who knew exactly what I wanted. My own sweet lovely strict man who could hurt me without hurting me.

Then he took me by the hand and led me down the corridor, put me back in bed, tucked me in.

'Now stay there.'

*   *   *

It is traditional to believe that an interest in punishment derives from the English experience of boarding school, but this, I'm afraid, is comfortable cliché. The boarding school that I attended between the ages of eight and eighteen was full of ponies and diplomats' daughters. Everyone had anorexia and took drugs but there wasn't an evil nun in sight. Discipline, such as it was, was detention, in the form of cleaning and running. I was good at running, in every sense of the word.

I didn't think about sex until my final year when we staged *Romeo and Juliet* and for some reason I was playing the latter. There was a weed from Eton playing Romeo, in whom I couldn't have been less engaged. In rehearsals, however, a certain Martin Finn threw himself into the role of the firm father Capulet, and, finding his daughter in love with the wrong man, dealt me a blow that was way beyond any suggestion made by the author.

'Hey,' I said, cheek stinging, 'you're supposed to threaten, not hit.'

'Oh,' he said. 'Never mind, I thought I would pull your hair as well.'

I fell in love with him immediately and we enjoyed extended periods of relentless kissing in the art department, to which I had the key, being a favourite of the art master, who was the only person I had ever listened to.

Martin Finn wanted to be a professional actor so he did not mind being instructed to exhibit his talents. It was not Martin in whom I was interested (he was from Kent) but the strict Capulet – thank you, Shakespeare. I had not discovered Petruchio at that point. That perfect hero arrived for A levels and inspired me to take the exams required to study English Literature.

So I directed Martin Finn and he stayed in character. It was lucky he didn't have a sense of humour and was unimpeded by self-consciousness as it meant he took the drama very seriously. So I fucked for the first time, surrendering to the energy of this seventeen-year-old father, who held me down on the floor, sat astride me and pinned my hands down in the dust. My summer dress went up above my waist. My thighs, bare, became filthy as the moist skin squirmed in the chalk and dust from the kiln. Capulet, getting his hands dirty, rubbed them in my face and then kissed me quite hard and without any pretence of affection. He was enjoying himself.

The mechanics were dick and cunt. He didn't know how to arouse me with his hands, but I didn't mind that. The words and the force had made me wet. I would have wanked if he hadn't fucked me, but he did fuck me, quite slowly for a beginner, which shows good instincts. He asked me if I was OK at one point, the Etonian taking over from Capulet for a minute.

I was OK. I was on my back on the floor with my legs over his shoulders and his wide dick plunging into me. He thrust himself into me, further and further, holding my arms down as he did so. I struggled. He held. He started to thrust to his own needs, bringing himself nearer and nearer to orgasm, forgetting me, but holding me down, and came.

Surprised by the force of his release, he grabbed my face and kissed me, very hard, but this time with the gratitude that is so often passion.

Martin Finn was pliable and appreciative. Standing up and looking over me, he stared with genuine respect at the sixteen-year-old Juliet, half naked, dishevelled, dirty legs spread over the floor, no knickers, hands in her bush.

'Did you come?' he asked.

'No. But I'm going to now.'

Capulet knelt down to watch closely as Juliet's slut hand disappeared into the place for which Shakespeare had so many entertaining metaphors.

'Three fingers?' he said

'Three fingers,' I agreed.

'I didn't know girls could do that.'

'We can have more than one. We can have as many as we like.'

'You're joking!'

'I'm not. I could have eight if I wanted.'

'Is this your first time, you know, all the way?'

'Yes.'

'I thought there would be blood.'

'Are you disappointed?'

'Of course not. What an extraordinary question.'

'Sorry. I don't know much about boys.'

We wrote to each other for a time. I used a Tempo pen and postcards of Alfonse Mucha pictures. It was the fashion to have a boyfriend, but then we lost touch. I spotted him in a period drama on the television some years later. He was not playing the stock Gothic hero that I would have predicted after his fine performance on the floor of the art department. He was playing one of those meek fraternal types that represent what the author sees as the correct moral direction.

The Capulet afternoon was the moment that the road bent and I began to travel down a path whose signposts pointed to perverse passion and peculiar pastimes.

Daddy always dressed me and promised that he would take me to Paris, to the shows, and buy me one thing that I wanted. Which was something to look forward to. Paris and Daddy. I could sit there in the front row with all the other prostitutes.

I had some expensive clothes that he had bought for me but which I didn't like much because he got furious when I spilt things down them. I didn't really see the point of

spending £1,000 on an outfit that you couldn't have fun in
– if they were ruined by a bit of grass or mud or come or
whatever. It was usually his fault anyway. He bought me
the stuff, then fancied me, then made me have sex in them.

I kept my clothes at Daddy's house – in a school trunk
with my name on it. Sometimes he told me to go and change.
He liked to watch me, half-naked, crouched over the trunk
throwing things over my shoulder to find the required item.
Then he would make me fold everything up and put it back.

You will be unsurprised to hear that he had very specific
tastes in what I should wear. He liked socks – to the knee
or ankle. He liked knee socks and a bare bottom and a neat
bush, or a bare one. He liked a short vintage tea dress, with
a demure collar, and flat strappy Mary Jane shoes. He didn't
like hats but he did like jackets that looked like blazers. He
liked my hair in little-girl styles – bunches, ponytail, braids.
He liked a tennis skirt, bare legs, plimsolls, no pants. He
liked grey culottes and a black bra. He loved a tight white
Aertex shirt.

Winter was short kilts and long socks or pinafore dresses
with polo necks and a ponytail and boots of varying length
and height. Nights were usually baby-doll pyjamas. He
didn't like anything that prevented easy access. So pencil
skirts were out, rather to my disappointment. All trousers
were prohibited except jodhpurs, which drove him mad. He
liked plain cotton knickers in white or black and nothing
else. He hated cheap Ann Summers stuff and clichéd
reader's wife crotchless or anything nylon. If it was going to
be sheer it had to be silk. He liked plain and pure with a St
Trinian overtone. I'm afraid a hockey stick was his idea of
heaven. Mine was tea, bath and bed. With good fucking in
there somewhere.

He liked a very short full dress, which barely covered the
top of the arse and sometimes showed my knickers when I

bent over. He enjoyed that Benny Hill view and had given me some old-fashioned frilly pants in order to enjoy it all the more.

I had range of high boots and shoes, which were difficult to walk in. Daddy liked me to struggle in them, wearing a short dress and no pants, so that when, for instance, I attempted to bend down to get in or out of his car, he could view my legs, pants and red face. Sometimes, if I was really struggling, he got to see my arsehole, which he enjoyed, as did I, giving him the full exposure and knowing I would give it to him whenever he wanted it and he would take it whenever he felt like it. I was consistently open. Open all hours. I had never experienced that before.

3. 1983

Daddy was particularly strict about food. I had never had conventional ideas about food. My grandmother only ate Ryvita and Marmite and drank what she described as 'gin and it', though I never discovered what the 'it' was. She drank particularly on Sundays and then went to church, sat in the front pew and yelled out requests for hymns while the vicar was giving the sermon.

Dogs always barked at her and I think that says a lot about a person. I sometimes felt like barking at her. Once I barked at Daddy and bit him and he made me stand with my face to the wall for an hour. Then he came up behind me and put his hand up me and found out how much I wanted him. He caned me. I came but I still wanted to bite him.

My grandmother drank rather than ate, but she had a strange relationship with bananas. I think because, as a child of the war, she had only ever eaten one, it had set up an obsession. There were always bananas in the house, great bunches of them, stacked in absurd pyramids in silver urns, dotted around the house, in the hall, for instance, and on the polished walnut sideboards of the dining room.

These embarrassing fruits were bought in bulk by the staff through an arcane economic infrastructure that I never understood. I was vaguely aware that it could not have been their own money that they were using to buy household items and food, but there were no overt transactions which explained their income.

Later, I discovered that my grandmother kept piles of cash around the house, as she kept gin bottles around the house, but in different places. Mrs Erin, the housekeeper, oversaw the cleaning, so she knew where everything was. Mrs Erin was an honest and moral person. She simply retrieved the money needed and accounted for it in an immaculately presented school exercise book.

I was amazed when I went to boarding school and discovered the existence of a ritual where people sat down at tables at designated times with portions on plates in front of them. Later, as a straying waif, I was adopted by various friends' parents and there were meals in their houses, though I was always concentrating on fulfilling the demands of manners rather than the food. I never knew what I was eating but I did know which fork to use and not to retain the butter knife for one's own purposes. When I lived in New York I ate when I was hungry, which wasn't very often on account of the cocaine.

So there I was, demented from Manhattan, chaotic lifestyle, a lot of fun but no self-control, and Daddy would make me sit down properly and eat what was put in front of me with no argument. If I was slow, he fed me and was quite capable of doing so in a crowded restaurant. I liked this, particularly when I was sitting in his lap. People stared. I was dressed like a teen geisha thanks to Daddy's business trips to Tokyo and his shopping trips around the Shinjuku.

Daddy liked to see me in a tight silk cocktail dress, slit up the thigh.

It was perfect, fitting into his lap, feeling his soft cotton shirt, the total of his protection, him stroking my hair and my neck with his big clean hands, smelling him. It was better than drugs and that's saying a lot. I would sit in his lap and he would make me eat fruit, or bits of chicken, or chips, or something more sophisticated. He would encourage me gently in my ear. 'You eat that, you're doing very well.'

I retrieved some lost part of myself.

Daddy said that every woman he had ever met had problems with food and he wasn't having it. 'It's no wonder they don't have any genuine power,' he said. 'All their time and energy is taken up with feeling ashamed of themselves.'

Now I am old and peri-menopausal and facing an array of incipient cancers and bone conditions, I have firm opinions about the politics of body image, the sources of subservience and the grotesque semiotics foisted on women by supercilious bullies in marketing departments. Now I am old and wise, I am ashamed of women who heedlessly perpetrate their own objectification without questioning it, thinking that, by collusion, they will service their own cheap desires, ignorant of the fact they are making a place where neither they nor anyone following their example will have any meaningful influence.

Daddy thought I had a thing about my weight, but he was wrong actually. When I thought about it, which wasn't often, I thought I was perfect. I didn't want to be taller or smaller or fatter or thinner. I was boyish in one way, but with enough breasts and arse to play about with if I (or anyone else) felt like it.

It wasn't the weight. I had flat stomach and chic ankles – still have actually. It was the way in which you were supposed to eat. I had a thing about sitting down in one place for too long. I liked to be on the move. I tended to get up from the table after about five minutes and it drove Daddy mad. He liked sitting for hours, doing what I don't know how to do: eating very slowly and talking.

'Stella. Sit down! You're going to finish that. If we have to go through this again, I will tie you to the chair. It's up to you. And don't you dare sulk.'

These scenes triggered delinquency and often I actually threw myself on the floor, screamed out loud and cried, like a B-movie demonic possession. Who knows what was lurking there in the depths, but my body would tremble and play out in the throes of catharsis. I have always had orgasms fairly easily, vaginal and internal, and I suspect my body was easily triggered to release stress. The meal-time scenes made me let go of some old-forgotten indescribable misery and rearranged the sensual wiring.

I began to have an appetite and I began to taste things. But only when I was with him. Only when I was safe and hungry and there was a delicious thing with a nice smell. I saw the point of his rules, though he hadn't considered their outcome, only their enaction. He liked the fact that they aroused me, he liked the sight of my smudged lipstick and sulky face and flushed recalcitrance and crossed arms. He liked the power. Screaming and screaming and screaming. How many men allow you to do that and remain unafraid and present and kiss you and fuck you?

Wasn't he just a sick old control freak? I hear you ask. I think not. I think he cared about me enough to want to teach me another form of sensuality, the sensuality of food. He certainly enjoyed it. He talked about it often enough. He knew a lot about it, having travelled all over the world. He told me he had eaten a guinea pig in China. With rice. 'They'll eat anything that moves over there,' he said.

He ate anything that moved over here as far as I could see. And shot anything that moved after 12 August. He wasn't beyond ordering pasta with a fig sauce. I only really like about five things, and confectionary makes up three of them. Once he found sweets in my bag and spanked me then and there. Then he threw them out of the window. I laughed because I imagined a packet of Opal Fruits landing on somebody's head, or on the ground in front of a delighted child. My bum was red, but I still laughed. That day, he hadn't hurt me that much. Just enough to arouse me.

'You're not smoking and you're not eating sugar. Get used to it.'

I clung to him, kissing him, feeling his erection pressed against me, desperate, pleading for him to fuck me.

'You must do as you are told, young lady.'

At times like this he would pull off my wet pants and rub me with his hand until I started to shake. Then, with his hands firm on my flesh, he would push me open so that the tongue of my clit was so exposed I could feel the air on it. Clothed, he would push himself hard and deep inside me and orgasms could subsume us both. I would be grateful and totally in love with him as our mouths melted into each other and I smelled his smell. The smell always has to be right. It just does. And Daddy's smell was right.

He made me eat things like scrambled eggs and smoked salmon. He ordered for me in restaurants. He glared me down if I argued. It was such a relief.

Eating is ugly. I had always thought it shouldn't be done in public. But I thought that having sex could be, so my ideas were schizoid, I suppose. I thought that popcorn should be banned in cinemas but making out should be allowed.

I once asked Daddy if he would like a blow job while we were in a NFT screening of *Vertigo*. He told me to be quiet and watch the film. I sulked at this rejection. After all, I was only trying to be intimate. Apparently you are supposed to achieve intimacy in loving relationships. I have never seen the point of this since any form of heightened erotic atmosphere relies almost entirely on the exact opposite. It is very difficult to want to fuck the familiar, as the divorce statistics continue to reflect.

Daddy, always on my case about food, noticed that I didn't know how to cook after seeing me place an open can of soup straight on to an electric ring.

'Right,' he said, 'that's enough of that. You are learning to cook!'

'Don't be absurd,' I said.

Real women don't cook.

But I did as I was told purely on the grounds that I didn't have anything else to do. It cost him £950 if you please.

I didn't say anything. It was his money and his business.

The cookery 'college' in South Kensington was a silly place, run by a woman of about 48 with blow-dried blonde hair, Gucci shoes and a boss eye. She was polite and hard. She was also socially ambitious, knowing far too much about the land-owning families of England and making the most of her 'education' at Heathfield. She accurately described herself as 'Miss Charlotte'. She always wore navy blue, sometimes the hair was pulled off the face by a velvet hairband, the shirts were always ruffled at the collar. She wore a frosted pink lipstick that did nothing for her. She lived in Earl's Court and she pretended that she knew more about 'Lady Di' than she was letting on.

I do not know if she knew anything about food or not, because I did not. But Daddy looked at her 'prospectus', perused the recipes and announced himself to be satisfied. 'I look forward to tasting the fruit fool,' he said.

'You're a fruit fool,' I muttered.

'What did you say?'

'Nothing.'

The pupils, if that is the correct word, were expensively ill-educated Sloanes who had just left school and were preparing to get married.

'Do you hunt?'

'Where do you ski?'

'Where does your father live?'

'Do you know the McNair-Campbells?'

'Did you come out?'

There was one gay young man called Peter who had come out in the non-debutante sense of the word. He had been sent there by his rich older lover who, rather like Daddy, felt that the spoiled (but beautiful) young consort should be armed with some useful skills. Peter turned up in a major pinny on the first day, became hysterical at the mention of Fanny Craddock and we hit it off immediately.

We worked together on station three and I have to admit that Peter carried me. He was more nervous than I was, more willing to please and less willing to waste his lover's money. He genuinely wanted to be able to make perfect choux pastry and plait cheese bread. I genuinely did not. I wrote 'fuck off' in felt pen on my white hat. Jesus Christ. I had seen The Stranglers at Hammersmith Palais.

Miss Charlotte's reaction to this was to look at me with a repellent pretence of affection and then say politely, 'I'm afraid I'm going to have to ring your father, Miss Black. I think it's unfair to waste his money and unfair on the class to be disrupted, don't you? They are paying for lessons and they are trying to learn even if you are not.'

Miss Charlotte thought Daddy was my real father and he had supported this delusion by making me wear clothes that made me look about sixteen. I didn't wear make-up to school. My hair was in bunches and he had bought me innocent-looking but short pinafore dresses, which I was forced to wear with Liberty-print blouses, knee socks and strappy flat shoes. My dark fringe was as long as that of a Shetland pony.

Miss Charlotte made him come and pick me up. He had to beg her to let me stay. Daddy, for his own entertainment, told her that I had had a very troubled background, that my mother had died and that he had had to bring me up on his own. He knew he'd done a bad job, but he was a man alone. If only he'd had somebody who was as good a teacher as Miss Charlotte.

I had my finger down my throat but Miss Charlotte bought it. She definitely fancied Daddy, which I could understand, and thought in some recess of her Sloane synapses that if she allowed me to stay she might get a dinner out in a Fulham Road bistro, or something.

I thought he was going to punish me in front of her. Over the knee, skirt up, bare behind, hard hand, there and then, in her room. It would have been worth it – she was so straight, so repressed. It would have been interesting to see the amazement on her face. But he and I both knew it wasn't worth the risk. We knew that pervery must be played in subtle ways and that the rules of complicity were often obscure to the point of invisibility.

He drove me home to Cheyne Walk without saying a word. I looked out the window and chewed gum. I didn't care if I went to Miss Charlotte's or not. I didn't care if I could cook or not. I wondered what the new Cure album was like.

In the hall he turned me round, unzipped the navy-blue pinafore dress and said, 'Take off your clothes.'

I pouted but did as I was told and stripped for him, allowing the dress to fall off me and onto the ground. I stepped out of it and unbuttoned my shirt from the front, showing him my erect nipples. I left my white knickers and white knee socks on.

'Everything,' he said, pushing his fingers into the elastic of my pants and pulling them down to my feet with one strong and swift movement.

I stepped out of the small cotton pool and peeled my socks off.

'Fold everything up, put them on the chair over there and stand in front of the mirror.'

I did as I was told and stood regarding my naked self in the pier gilt mirror. I could see my face, breasts, belly, thighs, but not down to my feet. The light was such that it cast a golden glow, making me more rounded than I in fact was and reflecting back the face of a girl/woman who was not ready to take on the mask of the latter. I don't think I could be described as beautiful in the conventional sense of symmetry and bone structure, but I have presence, great skin, good 34C round tits with small brown nipples and dark-lashed dark-blue eyes, which flash with anger and mockery, one as easily as the other. My mouth is quite full and red and swells into a pout as easily as it smiles. I liked what I saw.

'Stand there until I give you permission to move,' said Daddy.

So I stood in the hall in front of the mirror with an umbrella stand and a portrait of a man with a gun and a dead pheasant. He hung his coat up and disappeared into the house for what felt like hours. The wet ran down my leg, as I looked at myself in the mirror, naked, wondering what was going to happen to me.

After a time I felt hungry and I wanted sex. Soon I didn't know what I wanted more, a piece of toast with Marmite or his dick.

I received neither. He returned to the hall, slapped me once, very hard, on the right buttock, so that his red fingers could be seen staining the white flesh. Then he told me to go bed, which I did, without sex or food or anything. I was made to read my book until he came and turned the lights out.

I spent the next half an hour lying on top of the cover, naked, legs spread, fingers way up myself, bringing myself to orgasm and moaning out for him as I did so. I called and called and came and came, everything twitched and wanted. But he did not appear. It was a new punishment. Abandonment. Withdrawal. Control. He knew what I wanted and he wouldn't give it to me. It was torture. Torture without physical pain, without the sharp excruciations with which we usually played. My whole body wanted him.

I was still wet in the morning when, half asleep, I came round to a creeping feeling of intense dissatisfaction. This was slowly but surely blocked as his erection entered full and forceful from the back. He fucked me slowly and for a long time, silently, pushing himself into me again and again, as I widened and widened and received him, groaning with the pure pleasure of simple entrance and simple sex. Still curled behind me, he came, breathing his relief into my hair and neck and, as I joined him, I realised that I must and would do anything for him. I also realised that I never wanted to leave him. And this, for reasons I could not fathom, made me want to cry.

He told me to get up and make breakfast.

'What about Susan?'

'She has an appointment this morning. Make breakfast, please, and don't argue.'

I might have argued but for the fact that, at that moment, I was completely in love with him and wanted to please him. Also, I was starving and risked not having anything to eat if I didn't provide it. So I clattered around in the kitchen and made an omelette, which incorporated a haddock, sauce Mornay and Gruyère cheese.

Daddy said it was delicious, kissed me and drove me to school. On the way, he told he told me to behave myself because the class was expensive and he would have to pay for it even if I did not attend. Daddy, like many rich people, did not believe in wasting money. He was quite capable of spending £3,500 on an armoire and then quibbling about the delivery charge being incorrect to the tune of £1.50. I obeyed him, despite the compulsion to kick Miss Charlotte in the middle of her smug shins.

For the rest of the course he would pick me up at the end of lessons at 3.30 p.m., to stop me going to the wine bar with Peter, I suppose, and would ask me questions about what I had learned. I had to show him my recipe book.

'What's this?'

'It's what's happening to Aries this month.'

'Oh for God's sake.'

Daddy was a Virgo and therefore did not believe in astrology, which didn't stop him being a classic Virgo.

One Thursday afternoon he said, 'Right. Tomorrow is Susan's day off. I want you to make me the baked cod with horseradish sauce and tartare sauce. I will also have chocolate mousse. Susan can buy the ingredients today.'

I flushed slightly. I wasn't completely confident, having giggled all the way through the lessons. I had to cook the meal and serve it. I had never cooked a meal in my life let alone served anything. Miss Charlotte had delivered various extraordinary lectures about 'flatware presentation' and the indispensability of a hot plate, but I hadn't paid any attention.

Daddy's idea of the appropriate costume for this particular evening was a small white apron with a pie-crust frill and a tiny blue short-sleeved dress, which he bought in Denny's. It was an authentic oufit, of the type worn by maids in hotels, and he found some tight pale-blue cotton pants to go underneath. They were slightly small, making my buttocks look rounder and creeping up and into various crevices, which was both annoying and stimulating.

My legs were smooth, bare and brown. The slingbacks were white and pointed, as were the remarks muttered under my breath as I fiddled about in his kitchen, turning all the ovens on at once because I didn't know which switch pertained to which bit of the cooker, didn't know and didn't care. So I just fired everything up and got the gas rings going and lit cigarettes off one of them. I then poured myself a glass of champagne and wandered around looking into cupboards. There were whisks and openers and the various appliances that had become familiar at station three and were to do with roux and rolling.

For reasons best known to himself, Daddy chose not to supervise me, which was a big mistake. I did try. I really did. I extricated chopping boards and knives and mixing bowls. I got everything out. There was a lot of banging and crashing and squinting at my handwritten recipe book which was unhelpfully scrawled with shoe shop addresses and suggestions about after-school activities to Peter.

I opened the page to the prescribed cod dish and discovered a picture of a shark rendered in blue Biro and illustrated with a leg in its mouth. There were some cryptic clues numbered from one to five, which seemed to have something to do with the intended course but were difficult to decipher.

I sat down, fiddled about with my Sony Walkman, smoked another cigarette and wished that the ingredients would somehow sort themselves out, divide themselves up into the various courses and make their own decisions about seasoning. A potato rolled off the table and banged onto the floor. It was obviously trying to escape, so there was hope. Perhaps the bags of flour would fuck off out of it as well.

I had no idea what I was doing. He had paid £950 and I didn't know if I was supposed to take the grey bit off the cod or not, or how much butter to use with the sauce since I had not written down any measurements. Cod moves in mysterious ways. I laughed to myself and eased myself easily into a second glass of champagne.

The third glass of champagne pushed me from insouciant and cheerful to mawkish morbidity and I began to resent not having a mother. I didn't usually mind this, as, in general, they are overrated and I didn't really see the point of them, but suddenly if I had had a mother there would be somebody to ring up and ask for advice about what to do with gelatine. Read a cookery book might have been a sensible suggestion, but sense has never been my métier. I tended to do what felt right and hoped for the best. Suddenly I was subsumed by a feeling of self-pity and loneliness. I was small and helpless in a grand kitchen full of equipment whose attributes were unconnected with any identifiable use. I was back in the school art department, mixing things for the sheer pleasure of assessing consistency and their potential as a material to make form. The result, in the case of the so-called chocolate mousse, was a gelatinoid substance that brooked no order and seemed to be of little use to man or mammal. It was, however, the correct colour.

I knew from the start that Daddy was going to be impossible.

The tomato soup was too salty. The vegetables were overdone. The bread was too damp.

I walked in and out of the dining room where he was sat like an oligarch at the head of his long table, waiting to be served on some unnecessarily valuable china that he had spent hours acquiring from salesrooms.

'This is revolting,' he snapped, as I dropped a plateful of limp beans down in front of him.

For the first time since I had known him his face looked ugly. His mouth was tight and cruel, his teeth were old and grey. I hated him. I hated him and I hated men and I hated women for cooking for them and looking after them and forming an unnatural cultural history where service was expected.

By the time it came to the chocolate mousse, I was furious. The chocolate mousse was more successful because it is relatively simple and it is full of chocolate in which I am quite interested. I ate a huge amount of it in the kitchen before ladling it into a cut-crystal dish and decorating it with cream from a specialised bag, as suggested by the Miss Charlotte technique of home-making.

I was flushed and stressed and pumping with a sugar rush. I had food all down my front and chocolate all over my face and I had broken a nail so far down the finger it had turned red and was throbbing. Cooking was not my art and it never would be. I would never be interested and that was all there was to it. There were places to go and people to meet. And I'd had enough of him sniffing the stuff and wincing and looking disappointed.

'Stella,' I heard him call, 'where's the pudding?'

I walked in, walked up and dropped it on his head.

The dish stayed on his head then slid off and smashed onto the parquet floor. Chocolate ran everywhere. Down his face, down his collar, down the front of his shirt, onto the table mat in front of him. A river of brown oozed over the hunt in full cry. I know clowns throwing pies isn't funny, but I have to say that this was, and remains one of the most satisfying experiences of my life.

He did not retain his dignity and nobody could have. His face was covered in mousse and there was a mint leaf in his hair. I wondered if I should go and hide. There was going to be real trouble. I thought he might expel me out of his life – many men would have done, after all. I might have crossed some invisible line, a line bordered by his manly pride. I don't think he was expecting this, and it did come as something of a shock. He had never genuinely lost his temper with me, being a calm person, stern and silent rather than volatile and passionate. He was quite gentle really when it came down to it. But this. He was covered in pudding and ignominy. If he had done this to me I would have gone mad.

I stood transfixed.

He stood up, walked over to me, chocolate splattering onto the floor as he did so. I thought he was going to slap my face and I moved out of his way. He grabbed me and kissed me so that I was covered in the chocolate as well.

Then he took my wrist and marched me to the bathroom.

He pushed me into the shower, still in my 'uniform'.

He pulled it off and threw it out of the curtain and onto the bathroom floor. He was harder than I had ever seen him. I knelt down, the water pounding down on my head and face, and I sucked him. I wanted to attend to him, to apologise, actually, as I had lost control. I sucked and licked until he lost it and came, the white liquid spurting onto my breasts and washing away down the plughole with the last remnants of the chocolate mousse.

I stepped out of the shower smelling of soap. I was warm and clean and up for anything.

'You do not deserve this,' he said as he pushed my legs behind my shoulders and fucked me on the bathroom floor.

At the end of 1983 I spent Christmas with Daddy. Christmas, of course, is ghastly and I have never met anyone over the age of twelve who does not loathe it. It is a festival for which nobody has voted, representing a deity in which few believe and providing accurate resonance of essential misery. Try as I might, I could not forget the seasons of the past where the ritual had been managed by my grandmother and I would have been better off in care. Christmas taught me to have no hope. It also taught me to expend no energy in the wanting of material things, because the 'presents' were items wrapped in loo paper that she had found at 3 a.m. on Christmas Eve and had been removed from the downstairs loo. There was a tree because it was organised by Mrs Erin, but the only decorations on it were made by me out of cardboard and glue and glitter.

My grandmother veered between lurid descriptions of Santa, whom she painted as a cross between a paedophile and a burglar, and hysterical proclamations about how lovely everything was. I became less unhappy when I stopped expecting anything.

When I was very young and confused I would ask her if my father was coming to get me for the holiday to which the reply would be, 'He's dead, dear, so he can't.' I didn't actually know what dead meant for some time so I didn't understand the reason for what I saw as his disapproval of me personally.

One takes everything personally as a child. I didn't grow out of that until I was at least thirty. Everything was about me. Daddy would tell me that everything was not about me and, though I understood the reasoning, I never really believed him. It just didn't feel true. On the one hand he tried to tell me to grow up, but on the other he treated me like a child and wanted me to stay that way because it excited both of us, and because he knew where he was and he knew the more he succeeded in this area the less likely it would be that I would leave. I think he dreaded being left.

His wife had left him by dying. I never got to the bottom of his mother, but I suspect she had a lot to answer for as most mothers do. As Quentin Tarantino said, they're not called mothers for nothing.

Daddy was right to be nervous as I was prone to spontaneous departure. I believed in escape and had never seen anything wrong with it. I just went. I once left a boyfriend in the middle of lunch. He was about to fork into an apple tart and I went to Delhi. I had left Granny's house by the time I was sixteen and, angry, I did not reconnect with her just because telephone companies suggested it during peak advertising time.

I wasn't angry just because of Christmas, by the way, but more because she kept getting drunk and insulting me. There is only a number of times that one can be described as a 'slut' before one looks at the train timetable. It wasn't a formal departure but a casual journey from which I did not return. I took the sponge bag but left most of the shoes. I sometimes wondered whether she had noticed. I wrote to her to tell her that I was going to university and that the trustees were springing money for a flat. I received an education and I wasn't likely to starve to death. Then I went to New York and spent happy Christmases in Connecticut with various mad people, who laughed and took drugs.

Daddy's parents were dead. They had died at mature ages and he did not seem to be traumatised by the fact beyond a kind of secret and sensible sadness that did not subsume him. He knew how to enjoy himself and did actually say, 'Ho ho ho.' There was a tree which took three men to lift into the hall of the Cheyne Walk house. Susan stood on a ladder for a day with gold balls and tinsel. The lights glittered and winked with authentic grotto glamour as I worried about what to buy my lover and, unable to make any useful decisions, bought fifty things of varying unsuitability. He opened them all up with surprise and delight and I loved him for that, realising that he would not have been seen dead wearing a tie with birds on it.

My surprise and delight were genuine particularly when a lumpy stocking was placed on the bed. Jewels. Shoes. Clothes. Books. Toys. Underwear. Everything was right. He was laughing and I was full of glee and love and egg-nog.

It was the first Christmas I had ever had that followed middle-class convention. I was aware, from information received, that 25 December carried certain predictable receptions for most people and now I was one of them. I felt safe. I started to relax and, as a result, I became slightly hysterical with excitement. I felt all my dreams were coming true. I was going to stay in love with this wonderful father person until I dropped down dead. I was destined to be secure and loved. He guarded my future and everything in it and it would all be all right. It was the egg-nog, I expect, or the sherry, or youthful naivety or pure transference. Experience had not taught me about the reality of the future. Daddy was God the Father, all seeing and all powerful and I started to meld into him, letting myself go as one might let oneself out of an aeroplane with a parachute.

'I love you, Daddy.'

'I love you too, darling.'

I never thought for one minute that our relationship was wrong, let alone dysfunctional. He was the parent who set the moral code and whose decision-making could be relied upon as being correct and sensible. I did not think I was particularly different to anyone else. I thought there were a lot of daddies out there but I had been lucky enough to find a great one. It was only later that I discovered there are not a lot of daddies out there, but a lot of sons seeking mummies. Daddies are thin on the ground, particularly

Daddies who not only have innate strength, generosity and a sense of themselves, but can play with pain and scenes without being abusive.

We spent Boxing Day in bed. He bound my wrists behind my back with tinsel, which was a seasonal touch. Then he made me eat a mince pie, which I hate, so I spat it out on the floor. I had to stand with my face to the drawing-room wall with a red arse for that. Christmas red. He made me stand for half an hour, though during this period he would stand behind me and stroke my tits and the back of my neck and my throbbing buttocks until I nearly went mad.

We spent New Year apart. He said duty called and he had to mingle with grown-ups. I suspected he meant the parents of his late wife, but I didn't want to know the details. I went and sulked in my flat for a bit, then rang up a group of queens and told them the champagne was open. We did a lot of dancing and arguing about whether fur was right or not. On New Year's Day we all put on hats and had tea at the Ritz.

I told them about Daddy and they didn't think it was pervy, but queens never think anything is pervy. They are sophisticated like that and it was the 1980s. Everyone was waking up to the delights of perviness. They told me there were clubs where you could get whipped and more. There was one with a bath in it and a person could get pissed on by strangers.

Pissed on? I hadn't thought of that. It seemed like a good idea. I suggested it to Daddy, who wondered who should do the pissing, but liked it because it was filthy. In the end he lay naked in an empty bath and I pissed on his face. It made him hard. It was the first moment when I had taken the dominant position. I liked it because it was new, a naughty novelty, and it aroused him, which was nice. But if there was pissing to be done, I preferred it when he made me go to the loo and watched me.

4. 1984

I did not like Daddy's friends. They were wankers.
I was always on my worst behaviour because they
bored me and patronised me and doubtless laughed at
Daddy behind his back for being so stupid as to hook up
with a demented baby doll. They assumed I was after his
cash.

'So, Stella, what do you do?' they would say.

'Him,' I would reply, indicating our host.

People would occasionally ask me about the career that I
had pursued after I left Oxford. The dreadful answer was
that I went to Manhattan, took drugs, hung out with Keith
Haring, took drugs, had sex and went to clubs in the East
Village. I had private means. I pottered. I just was, which
you could be in the East Village, thanks to the legend of
Edie and the Warhol stars. You could just be fabulous.
Nobody asked you what you did as long as you were
photographed and seen and wore wigs. I was photographed
and seen and wore wigs. I did not feel the necessity to do
more than this. I watched and was watched. I lived in a

walk-up on 3rd and B. I was not ambitious. I hung out. I met Philip Glass. I waved at Quentin Crisp in the street. I went to Talking Heads concerts. Psychokiller. It was enough.

Daddy often told me off for being rude. 'You were very abrupt with Sylvia.'

'She was paralytic.'

'Don't answer back.'

'She believes in the death sentence, did you know that?'

'Sshh.'

'Well.'

'Eat your toast.'

'I don't like it. Was she one of those women who married Oswald Mosley?'

'Don't be ridiculous. She's forty-three years old!'

'That's what she says.'

'She is a very well-respected interior designer.'

'Yeah. I bet the lampshades are made out of human skin.'

'If you don't finish that now you'll go to bed. Do I make myself clear?'

It wasn't a frightening threat in the light of the fact that I always did want to go to bed, either by myself to read, or with him to enjoy his beautiful cock.

Sometimes he told me that he was going to punish me in front of his guests, but I knew he wouldn't do it. That kind of scene was found in erotic novels only, or some black-and-white fashion photographs. I relished the fantasy of Daddy dominating me in front of his absurd cronies but the reality would have been hell. Their level of sexual sophistication was sniggering about the memory of each other's stag nights in Annabel's. I told a man named Andrew that Daddy put me over his knee if I was naughty and he started sweating profusely. I thought he was going to have a cardiovascular episode. After that he kept asking me out for lunch but

Daddy wouldn't let me go. Most of his friends were red-faced, fat and fascist. They drank heavily to forget their debts and the fact that their trophy wives were tarnishing with age and there was nothing they or anyone could do to restore the polished veneer that had been so attractive at a hunt ball. Early 1980s, surgery was not what it is now. People tended to stick to their own tits and age group.

The Europeans were slithery and multilingual. Daddy and they shared some past history of skiing in Klosters or sailing on yachts around Porto Ercole. They wore an air of entitlement that was as irritating as their aftershave. The Europeans were more informed and more decadent, but they were sexist and therefore not sexy.

They were a dull mélange and I did not wish to engage with them on any level. I don't think Daddy was very discriminating in his choice of companion, present company excluded. He was strangely passive in his social choices and consequently flotsam floated onto his shore and stayed there, bedraggled and unshapely and providing no enhancement to the natural beauty of the environment.

When I teased him about it he would say they were his 'old friends' as if that was explanation enough. I, being in my twenties, did not have old friends in any sense of the word, and did not, as I do now, appreciate their value. I had new friends who were up for anything and occasionally died in car crashes. It was more important that they were fun than they were loyal or compassionate or resilient to my defects. I know differently now, of course, but then I could not understand why Daddy remained loyal to old bores. Sometimes I wondered if he was an old bore but decided he was English and public school and left it at that. He seemed to have missed most of the 1960s. I think he was making money. He liked musicals and made me go to *Oklahoma* where I saw Peter and his boyfriend and we screamed in the foyer.

'The campest thing I have ever seen,' Peter said. 'And that is saying something.'

'Daddy sings the songs in the shower,' I confessed.

'Are you sure he's straight?'

I didn't have to go to Daddy's shooting or fishing weekends, which was a relief as they sounded like hell. I rarely turned up to his soirées and drinks and dinners and, indeed, I was not invited to them unless there was another 'young person' and they wouldn't have anyone to talk to. Luckily the other young person was rarely as bad as his or her parents, though they tended to be confused and subdued. Inherited wealth can do that to a person. They hadn't begun to address the issues of money and love and control. They were living up to expectations that were not their own. They had no idea who they were or what they wanted. They liked me because I was insouciant and daring and looked like nothing they had ever seen. The girls were confined to demure cocktail dresses, I was in prom-girl net, stilettos and pearls, teamed with Viv Westwood twinsets. I did Edie earrings which I bought in second-hand shops and false eyelashes, which were difficult to find but worth the search. I had been influenced by *The Rocky Horror Show* and the gang girls in *Grease* and punk. They, well, the girls, had been influenced by their mothers and Diana Spencer.

I would make them sneak away with me and do my best to corrupt them. I was usually successful, especially with those who had received convent educations. They always had cannabis. We would go to the television room and smoke joints. Daddy had bought a video machine and, if we were lucky, we would be left alone to drink champagne and watch the mesmerising beauty of Al Pacino.

I would have to sit through dinner squashed between two middle-aged men who didn't know what to say to me and were too English to talk about relationships, particularly the one that they suspected I was having with their friend and about which they were undoubtedly jealous. Their wives were always in the room so they could never ask any of the questions whose answers they were keen to know. They did ask me how old I was fairly often and then say they thought I was younger with either a sense of disappointment or relief, depending on the nature of their inner life. Their wives were trickier and would have asked pointed questions in the drawing room after dinner if I had gone to the drawing room after dinner. I never made that mistake. I would sneak to the television room – a small study upstairs – with the other young person or persons, some of whom actually went and told their parents where they were going.

Daddy sometimes forgot about me during these evenings and I often spent them with his godson Stuart who was reading theology, if that tells you anything. Stuart admitted that he was probably a bit gay, but he did want to marry and have children. I told him that human sexuality was complicated and nobody should feel ashamed of that fact. They should be ashamed of violence and cruelty and paying for bad art, but not of the delicate hormonal balances with which they had been born and about which there was nothing they could do. They should embrace them and allow them and use them for pleasure. Otherwise one ended up miserable and repressed and probably sour, and what was the point? Well, that was my view. Stuart's only experience of life arrived from reading the *Spectator*. He could name the members of the shadow cabinet and talk about the diaries of Chips Channon but he knew nothing about sex. He made the mistake of listening to me. He was bright and sweet and effete and he had enough humour to make him worthwhile.

Once, Daddy walked into the study when I was sprawled about with a joint in one hand and Stuart's corduroyed knee in the other. The music, by The Specials, was loud enough to cause vibrations, but not, unfortunately for Stuart, loud enough to drown out my opinions.

'I think prostitution should be a legal service,' I was telling him, 'with regulated fees, medical supervision and a tax bracket. There is something to be said for it coming under the jurisdiction of the World Health Authority.' I was smirking smugly when Daddy walked in, all tall and fierce and Victorian – at his best in other words.

'Stella! Turn that bloody music down, it's making the floor vibrate.'

Stuart literally jumped to his feet and stood erect as if he was in the army.

'What do you think you're doing?'

I remained where I was, on the sofa, extremely relaxed and quite stoned. 'What does it look like I'm doing? I'm lying around talking to Stuart.'

Stuart started to stammer like a cartoon character. I don't think he had decided whether to be valiant and take the blame, or let me cop it. Certainly he did not have time to ask God what he thought.

Daddy knew who was to blame. 'What is that in your hand?'

'Nothing.'

'Stella, I can see it. Give it to me.'

'Give you what?'

'Stella!'

Daddy came up to me, took the joint out of my hand and flattened it in the Hermes ashtray. 'You're going to bed. Now.'

To Stuart's utter amazement he took me by the arm and dragged me out of the room.

I never saw Stuart again, but I did ask Daddy what he thought his godson must have thought.

'I have no idea what he thought,' Daddy said sternly. 'I expect he saw an insolent woman smoking illegal drugs in my house.'

'Well,' I responded, 'he had a hard-on.'

'I don't expect it will be his last.'

'Shall I fuck him?'

'No,' he said. 'I don't want you fucking anybody, thank you.'

'Am I allowed to with your permission?'

'I will not give permission. We're not bored yet, we don't need to swing, we need trust not risk. I don't want you fucking another man. If I decide to bring that element in, I will let you know. It may be a man, it may be a woman, but I will arrange it.'

'What if I don't fancy them?'

'You will.'

'Can I have a tattoo?'

'No. Now be quiet and finish that egg. I want to read the newspaper.'

I glared at him from underneath my fringe. 'I don't even eat breakfast. I told you that ages ago.'

'Stella! Do as you're told! And do not speak to me until you've finished. I mean it.'

He shot me a look that would have felled a telegraph pole.

I ate the egg and felt young. And wet. As usual.

One afternoon I went round to Cheyne Walk and found Daddy with an American called Daryl. He was talking a lot of rubbish so I assumed he was an artist.

I was right.

'I am interested in cultifying the commonplace presence,' he said. 'I want to be able to reproduce a suggestive atmosphere.' He studied my breasts with unembarrassed scrutiny. 'Symbolise it and by so doing neutralise it. I want to study the detachment of distortion and art's pathological enchantment with total retinality thus questioning whether the woman/object, addressed in an antithetical way, can achieve authentic non-objectivity. And . . . I wanna make a ladda money.'

Half of my face started to go to sleep as I contorted my muscles into a stiff pose designed to disguise boredom. Soon the features stiffened into a rictus as the blood ceased to oxygenate the vital veins. I looked at Daddy. He seemed to be convinced by all this flannel. I'm afraid he was easily conned in the realm of the arts. Too much Robert Ludlum and not enough Robert Hughes. He didn't know anything about twentieth-century art, but he had been advised to buy it by one of his interminable financial advisers. So here we were. Talking to an artist.

'I tell my students, it is axiomatic that my art must be about an objective relationship with vital forms that are Spinozan in their intellectuality. The breast, or the ankle, or the knee, reduced to mere geometry, can be made to represent a statement on the history of appropriation as well as man's inability to repress instinct. Or emotion if you will.'

On and on he went.

'And then there are all the dictums of abstraction, the questions of definition and irrelevance, of art and commerce, on inward decadence and outward religiosity. The question of whether the consolidation of universal concepts can be made through symbols, and whether the dequilibrated whole has a valid position in any universal principle or whether one must still provide the shock of fragmentation. This is complicated by the fact that in studying the female form we are hoping to empathise with the pre-Adamite, but we are also having to address the pleasure principle and all the Freudian machinery of understanding.'

'Of course,' said Daddy.

'Are you English?' Daryl asked me.

'Yes,' I said.

'I'm English on my grandfather's side. I'm Irish as well. And Australian. Where do your folks live?'

'They're dead.'

'Oh. You an orphan?'

'S'pose.'

'Were you in care?'

'No.'

'Oh. You have the look of a girl who has been remanded in custody.'

'You should meet my grandmother.'

Then he said, 'I would like you to model for me. Nood.'

'Why?'

'Well, honey. Your partner here has asked me to paint your portrait and, looking at you now, I see you have a lovely shape. It advertises anti-patriachal balm and it speaks to me. It speaks to me of radically different versions of natural illustrations; it tells me that it can help me to realise my Vision and help us to know that there is no such thing as uniform deification. Your shape, honey, your body, will represent Unawoman, the woman who can authenticate the important, indeed the life-giving contention that the universalisation of the organic aesthetic has destroyed all possibility of integrating the self which, as I am sure you will agree, has dangerous repercussions for all of humanity and to the progress of civilisation itself. You can help save us from this disintegration.'

I tried to be polite. But I knew that modelling would be boring and uncomfortable. I had known enough art students to know their trade in recumbent Venuses. I had, once or twice, made the mistake of trying to please them by divesting and subjecting myself to their stares and to long discussions about the traditions of design and whether birth control was responsible for the obsolescence of the fertility symbol as the great female icon and why, since then, the female icons had male bodies and why men liked looking at women and women liked looking at women.

These experiences had taught me that I was a tiny and almost useless part of their cause. They could utilise geometry, fad, the classical, training, matriachal nightmare or genuine talent, but they were not interested in reporting the nature of the model; to see me would confuse them. Their heads were full of concept and composition, the problems of tone, the pressures of modernity and their exhibitions.

I knew I would have to contort myself into some unnatural posture for hours on end and stare glassily and know that the mere blink of an eye would be seen as a seismic upheaval in the atmosphere of artistic concentration. I wouldn't be allowed to smoke or watch the television and I might have to pretend to eat cherries.

I am able to flatter myself and often do. I like attention but I do not need it in order to make me know my own beauty. I am not the Muse clattering up the stairs to the garret to be leered at by a dysfunctional lech with illustrative skills. The only reason I would have followed his tattered suit to his room would have been in order to avail myself of the laudanum that would doubtless have been on tap. Laudanum and syphilis. That was what the Muse could expect as payment.

I am not drawn to the distance created by Art Man. I am not interested in delving into his aura of secluded personal privacy. I do not see him as an interesting challenge or think that he might end up loving me and me alone. He is and always will be what used to be called selfish and is now called ego-based. He cannot connect. He is never present, unless he wishes to have sex, in which case he is in your face. When he speaks it is to expound for he cannot listen.

Art Man is never present.

I was not interested in Daryl's image of me except at the very basic level of fleeting entertainment because I knew it could never be me. Art Man painted, ate, painted. There was little pleasure involved in his scenarios. Sometimes he even forgot to offer you drinks.

'I am quite busy at the moment,' I lied.

'Aw,' he wheedled. 'Cam an. It won't take long.'

'I would like you to do it, darling,' said Daddy. 'I would like a portrait of you and I have commissioned Daryl to paint one as part of his forthcoming exhibition.'

Oh for God's sake, I thought. 'OK,' I said without enthusiasm, staring at the 'artist' with some dislike.

'God, they're worse than poets,' I told Daddy when Daryl had consumed his body weight in whisky and departed. 'Inauthentic sentiment wrapped up in narcissism.'

'Stella!' said Daddy. 'He's a very famous painter and his pictures go for fifty thousand pounds on the open market. Not only does this represent an investment, but it is an honour that he wants to paint you. You can do it for me!'

'S'pose.'

I found some gallery catalogues about Daryl and discovered that he had always painted nudes. Morose prostration was his métier. He understood flesh tones and was able to communicate auto-erotic self-sufficiency. His trick was to combine a photographic sensuality with a lurking sadism and this had found a market with collectors who appreciated the female form when it was rendered as debauched and defective. His *Ondine in Calipers* had recently fetched $90,000 in New York and his *Nymph with Her Eye Being Pecked Out by a Bald Eagle* had achieved acclaim at the

Venice Biennale. His skill was to disguise graphic inanity with sophisticated art-speak. He had stolen some of the more kitsch ideas from the turn of the century eroticists, combined them with a crude knowledge of mythology and decorated them with a considered intent to shock. His graduation show had featured a picture of Leda having anal sex with a swan and this had been made into a best-selling poster. Every feather had been painted with attention to texture and detail; the yellow beak of the swan could be seen entering the puckered button hole of the pleasured woman's arse. Daryl had not looked back.

He was possessed of graphic skills rather than the deeper and more complex capacities required by fine art but I'm sure he did not care. He was rich. He was getting away with it. Who could ask for more?

Daddy took me to the sittings because he did not want me to go alone.

'Don't you trust me?'

'No, I do not.'

'I don't even fancy that git.'

'He has a reputation for fucking his models. And I don't trust him not to hand out drugs. Most of the women in those pictures look stoned to me.'

'I thought they were supposed to be in the throes of ecstasy. Anyway what's wrong with the occasional joint?'

'I'm not arguing, Stella, you will do as I say. You're being painted, and I am taking you there. Anyway, I like staring at your naked body.'

'Fair enough.'

Daryl's studio was located in the middle of a network of alleys made of corrugated iron and wood and crowded with the contents of the inhabitants' lives. It was a huge 'space'. I mean a big loft with one wall of windows and filled up with old sofas, cacti, a bicycle, a fish tank, an old television, a wall of *National Geographic* magazines and a six-foot-high Native American totem pole tricked out with garlands of glinting fairy lights. Two naked male mannequins lay in a bath in the midst of a clutter of chicken wire, broken neon signs and shoes.

The Artist was wearing a white T-shirt and a pair of jeans that were authentically covered in paint. His art work was all about the place. Half-painted canvasses of moon-eyed women with luminescent skin tinged with greenish tones, big breasts and mannish hips. One, a bride, in the full white robe, had stabbed herself in the stomach and stared out, dying, as her intestines, realistically rendered, oozed from the middle of her body. The other hand was proudly showing her wedding ring. The title was *Rock*.

Daddy led me in by the hand and presented me proudly as if I was about to sing and play the piano. I looked up at Daryl through my fringe and scowled at him. I could scowl. It was the only exercise I took at that point in my life. Everybody else was doing Jane Fonda.

Daryl calmly studied me with his Art Man eye. This observation was supposed to look intelligent and intense, but was in fact a weird squint. I was wearing a short pair of navy-blue culottes, a sailor top and white plimsolls. Daddy had made me put my hair in a ponytail with a white ribbon. I had eyeliner and red lips and a look of utter contempt. This belied the fact that this adventure was beginning to excite me. I didn't know what was going to happen, and I was beginning to engage in the delightful prospect that is unknowabilty. Who needs prophecy? Daddy would take control. I was safe. I started to go with it. Daddy stroked my arse and I tingled. He could touch me and I wanted him.

'Daddy,' I whispered, 'can I bring myself off, please. I'm desperate.'

'No, you may not,' he snapped. 'Are you mad?'

Daddy was impressed by Daryl and, for reasons that I could not fathom, he felt the need to retain decorum in front of a serious artist. This showed how little he knew about either art or artists. I had had quite enough experience of them to know the one rule is to never take them seriously, at a personal level anyway, and to never allow them to make the rules.

'Are we going nood?' said Daryl as he busied himself with his sketchpad and pencils.

'What?' I said. 'All of us?' Perhaps I was going to be part of a threesome. Daryl and Daddy, Daddy and Daryl. I didn't fancy it much because I didn't fancy Daryl. He was too pretentious and too humourless, as Americans often are, I'm afraid, unless they are Jewish. However he carried himself as if he possessed a large dick and I would like to have seen it. Perhaps it was bigger than Daddy's. I smiled to myself.

'Just you, Stella. And stop being pert.'

'If she needs me to share her vulnerability I will go nood too,' Daryl offered.

'I don't think that will be necessary,' Daddy said politely. 'Arms up, Stella.'

I raised my arms above my head and Daddy peeled off the cotton top. I wasn't wearing a bra. Never did actually, unless I was told to. I unzipped the culottes myself. Daddy put his hands into the white cotton panties, groped my buttocks possessively, and pulled the pants down over my thighs and knees. 'Step out,' he said.

I stepped out.

Then I sat down and he knelt at my feet to untie my shoelaces.

'Good girl.' He kissed me on the lips.

Both men appraised me in my nudity.

'You didn't want her shaved?' said Daddy.

'Naw, I don't think so. Though it's a good look. A look I like, the bald pudendum. The pruned pulchritude of the innocent maiden, yeah, it's a look ah sure do like.' Daryl stepped into my personal space, knelt down on the floor, placed his face three inches away from my neat bush and stared at my mons as if he had left his glasses at home.

I looked down at the top of his shaggy grey head. I could feel the tip of his nose brushing against my labia and I wondered if he was going to put out his tongue and lick the tip of my clitoris. I could sense it beginning to twitch but not so that you could actually see this happening.

'Cute cunt,' he said. 'I'm tempted just to paint that. The vagina remains uncelebrated in art, ah believe. I'd like to redress that, perhaps do a series – old cunts, young cunts, bleeding cunts, dead cunts, cunts swollen with longing. Cunts with beards. Cunts with teeth. They are one of earth's great mysteries, after all. They are the closed doors of the great occult earth mother.'

I could see that Daddy was worried that he was going to end up with a carefully rendered portrait of my genitalia, which he would have some difficulty explaining to the various aged aunts who had promised to remember him in their multitudinous wills. Daryl remained kneeling with his face in front of my lower body then, without permission, he placed his hands on my vagina and pulled the lips apart so that he could see the internal folds. 'Well, honey, it is a flower.'

'Her face is lovely as well,' Daddy observed.

'She has the face of a witch child,' said Daryl. 'She is ageless and indefinable.'

He looked at my chest. 'And she has beeoodiful breasts. Not too big, not too small, perfectly proportioned.'

'I've never had any complaints,' I said primly.

'Go and lie on that sofa, honey, and I will arrange you.'

I lay naked on the sofa and surrendered myself to his control. There was a smell of turpentine and paint. I made myself comfortable, which was easy as there were a variety of velvet cushions. Daddy sat on a leather chair with a glass of red wine and observed with interest. I sprawled in the interests of provocation, stretching one leg over the back of the sofa and one towards the floor, so that he could see the lips of my mons opening up for him. I sucked my thumb, looked at him and gave him the child-adult. It was warm. I was naked. I was being watched by two men. I was beginning to enjoy myself. A familiar warmth started to ease itself around my pudendum and a smile arrived with it.

I wondered if Daddy had an erection. I hoped so.

Daryl sat in front of me and stared, waiting for an idea to stimulate his impeccable commercial instincts. I saw a man of about 53 with a fringe of grey-white hair, a flat nose and a compact body, which gave off an atmosphere of barroom brawl. He had Hemingway going on but I doubted he was the type to shoot himself.

'I wanted to paint you as Pasiphae,' he said. 'But I couldn't get a bull.'

'What do you mean?'

'She was the mother of the Minotaur, you know. He lived in the labyrinth and ate Athenians.'

I wished that I could eat an Athenian. I was starving and there was no sign of the chocolate cake that had been promised. 'I'm hungry, Daddy.'

'You'll just have to wait, darling. Daryl is working.'

Daddy had a respect for the artist because he didn't know anything about art. He did not know that its history described chicanery. He had the innocence of the person who is ignorant and thinks that if there is something outside his ken, there must be a reason for it. There must be some intellectual or mystical secret to which he had no access. Art for him was full of rules that he had not made and did not understand. He had a sense of beauty and a sense of sensuality, but he cared not a jot for anything after Rodin.

'Daddy, I'm starving! If I don't have something to eat I will faint.'

'Faintin's good,' said Daryl. 'The nymph dying of love; the fever of consumption; the spirit broken by cruel paternalism and domestic repression. Or perhaps an actual organic disease for which there is no known medicine – AIDS perhaps.'

I glared at him and was about to provide him with the full force of my (I like to think) effective vocabulary when Daddy said, 'God, you're a nightmare. What do you want?'

'What is there?'

'I think she better have something to eat, Daryl, or we will never hear the end of it.'

Daryl, stimulating himself in the warm comfort of his own art space, imagining, no doubt, that I was suffering from a terminal disease which he could paint, waved his paintbrush and said vaguely, 'Of course. I believe there are some things in the fridge, and a glass of wine.'

'She doesn't have wine,' said Daddy. 'She has a brown bread sandwich, some Marmite, a glass of Ribena and some fruit if she is still hungry.'

Some people might have been surprised by this eccentric decree, even unnerved. I of course wanted to fuck Daddy immediately because the food-control-protection drama triggered every single response in my body, as if he had put three fingers deep into me and found the nerve endings with which he had made himself so exquisitely familiar. The Art Man was faced with a young woman and an older man engaged in an arcane sexual subtext, but he hardly noticed. He wasn't interested. He was harvesting his vision; an anvil could have dropped on his head.

Daddy went over to the kitchen area of the studio and clattered about. He took his jacket off, which was a good sign.

Daryl arranged me like a toy. Eventually I ended up like the Boucher babe, on my front, arse up, face half turned to him. He quickly sketched me and then changed me again, putting me on my back, putting one leg behind my neck, so that my clit was forced to nip out and look around. The absurd position and the porno-exposure appealed to me. I was being controlled and watched. I was enjoying myself.

'You're very supple, honey,' he said, as he twisted my spine and rotated my neck like an owl. 'Do you do yoga?'

'No,' I said. 'It's probably the sex. I've had to do hundreds of different positions since I've been seeing Daddy. He's insatiable.'

Daryl looked impressed.

Daddy, buttering some bread, said, 'Stella! Behave yourself!'

Daryl smiled superciliously.

So did I.

'Ahm assuming he's not your real pop,' he said, 'though that sure has commercial possibilities.'

'No I am not!' Daddy exclaimed. 'Heaven forbid.'

'I have seen the world,' Daryl boasted. 'There's nothin' that can shock an artist. It is the gift of the artist to envelop all facets and aspects of life, to receive them, transmogrify them, tell them to the world for educative purposes. The artist must defy convention. It is his personal obligation and his private law.'

I rolled my eyes. We broke for lunch. Daryl had a beer and said that Baudrillard was right: incest was natural, that was why it was taboo. Daddy flinched, had a salad and handed me a sandwich. I sat nude at the table and ate it.

Both men looked at me: Daddy with affection, Daryl assessing the graphic possibilities.

'She sure has the Lolita thing going on,' he said appreciatively. 'I am reminded of Simone de Beauvoir's observations on La Bardot, "If they go astray, it is because no one has shown them the right path, but a man, a real man, can lead them back to it."'

'You must have a photographic memory,' I said.

'Ah sure do,' he said smugly, continuing to quote with the skill of a man accustomed to assiduous assessment and appropriation of other people's ideas. '"To spurn jewels and cosmetics and high heels and girdles is to refuse to transform oneself into a distant idol." You have that goin' on, honey, that and a dancer's body and a delightful bosom. You are free and wild. I lerv your indifference, your naivety, your goddamn arse – I'd like to see you dance . . . barefoot. How old are you anyway?'

'She is twenty-five,' Daddy said quickly.

'But young for my age,' I explained.

Daryl whistled. 'You sure are.'

'How old did you think I was?'

'I don't like to say, hun, but young. Too young.'

If I had been drunk I would have danced but, as it was, I went back to lie on the sofa. 'Daddy,' I whined, 'Daryl's in my fanny. He's looking right up it!'

Daddy stood up and came over to me. Looking down at me he said, 'Daryl is in charge, Stella. If he needs to look then he will look. If you close your legs I will smack you until you open them.'

'Ah, the slap,' said Daryl perking up. 'The red mark of patriarchal dominance. The woman beaten. The shrew tamed. The decadent crimson stain on white flesh.'

I could see that there was a real danger of them both getting carried away and I would be painted with a flaming arse.

Daryl looked at the red range of paints on his palette. 'Red on white,' he muttered. 'Punishment, I like it. It's got the resonance of the zeitgeist – could be the symbol of the failure of manhood The last desperate action of a fading gender. It's honest. It's beautiful!'

Here we go, I thought. Any excuse.

Daryl, who had assumed a certain range of rights for himself, told me to 'Lie face down, honey.'

He then slapped my buttocks a couple of times to assess the effect of his hand on my skin. He did it a couple more times.

'Very nice,' Daddy said. 'Lovely colour. But could be redder.' So, of course, Daddy delivered a few more swipes with his expert hand until I was yowling and flushed and both men started to become glazed and breathless.

'Ow! Daddy, I haven't done anything wrong!'

'You will.'

'Uh-huh,' said Daryl and stroked my glowing behind. 'We're getting there, I think.'

He then turned me over, lay me on my back, put one leg over my shoulder and one of the back of the sofa.

'The maenad with the broken back,' he explained.

I put my fingers in my cunt.

'Not now, honey.'

'Stella, do as you're told.'

The work took six months. I couldn't believe it. I thought it was never going to end. It was as if Dante had invented a new place from which the tortured spirit was never allowed to emerge.

Daddy was patient. He enjoyed the visits, but he always felt comforted by routine and repetition. He listened to the same symphonies and sometimes read the same books.

Daryl meanwhile treated me to the full range of his opinions. If Daddy had given permission I am sure Daryl would have fucked me and, sometimes, I wondered what it would be like if he did. I didn't believe in the sanctity of monogamy – monotony I called it – but I obeyed Daddy's rules in this department because I didn't want to lose him or hurt him. He had tamed me enough to ensure my compliance with this. I did as I was told. I flirted with everybody but I did not deceive him or make out behind his back. He was jealous and possessive and he did not want anybody else touching me. I enjoyed this but I did not test it. He had set the boundary and I was aroused enough by the boundary to fall in with it; I did not need to cross the boundary in order to find out if that would be more exciting.

I tended to leave the sessions wanting sex, but it was always Daddy who gave it to me.

I ended up as a nine-foot triptych! I was huge! Huge and naked. Daryl had painted three aspects and, though they were unforgivably superficial in their rendition, they contained some photographic truths – the three Stellas were defiant, bored and humble. They were all naked, all white, and they all rendered me at my most youthful – that is there was no sign of the twenty-something girl about town. There was a naughty nymph with no hips, teetering on adolescence and made 'romantic' by Daryl's immaculate attention to detail and his shameless sentimentalism. The eyes – I hesitate to describe them as mine – were slightly more moist than they should have been, the tendrils of the pubes were delicate and curled, the little lips poked through, a slight slit of red painted small but lewd.

The gallery was delighted. The PR girl told somebody that I was Daryl's illegitimate daughter and the oxygen of controversy propelled the show into the mainstream press. Daryl talked like a catalogue and everybody listened with respect. Daddy gained much pride and pleasure from seeing his girl portrayed to the public at large.

We hung around at the opening, which was a crush of people who had dressed up to come out. Daryl had other subjects on display but the paintings were smaller and attracted less attention from the hoi polloi – though the critics scrutinised them quite closely, squinting with their noses pressed close and then remaining silent. Most people stared at me – well, the picture of me – naked. This was nearly as good as if I had been naked, in that, by proxy, I received the kind of prurient attention that has long aroused me. I like being stared at, I just do. People stared at the picture of me and I stared at them staring at me. And I stared at myself. There was a lot of staring going on. Everybody talked about the paintings and aired their received opinions but nobody talked to me. And nobody recognised me.

'It's Daryl's new model, apparently she's related to him.'

They fucking wish, I thought.

'Really. How old is she?'

'God knows.'

'He's a genius.'

'Apparently Melvyn Bragg is here.'

'How much is it going for anyway?'

'It's been bought apparently. Private commission.'

Daddy paid Daryl £25,000 for the picture. I asked him where he was going to put it and he said he had no idea. I thought it was money very badly spent, but I did not say anything. It was his money. He obviously had enough of it to throw away, despite Africa.

'I think it's beautiful,' he said. 'The critics think so too and they should know.'

'Nobody has asked my opinion,' I muttered sulkily.

Daddy enjoyed his 'art' experience. In particular, everyone staring at the pictures of his naked Stella. His chattel was being admired without the danger of having to actually protect it. He left the opening with an erection. Jimmy drove us home and Daddy couldn't wait. I wasn't wearing pants so all he had to do was flip up my little black dress (Chanel – he had bought it for me for the opening) and give me a seeing-to there and then, in the back seat of the car. The Chanel dress around my waist, black stilettos still on my feet, I spread my legs for him. He pumped into me, keeping his mouth on my mouth, coming in great loud shuddering gasps.

'I love you,' he said.

5. 1984–5

I wondered whether I would marry my 'father', whether we would end up together. I didn't fancy silent breakfasts and the mundane detail of morbid domesticity. In the end, he read Robert Ludlum and Dick Francis and was obsessed about his health. And he had the rich man's lack of understanding for those unlike himself. He did not understand the power of £10 to a person who has nothing.

He had manicures and phantom tumours. He didn't like watching television and genuinely disapproved of it. He complained about programmes that he hadn't even watched. I asked him once if he had graduated from Cambridge with a degree in pomposity and he sent me out of the room. He had faults and I didn't want to have to think about them let alone live with them. I didn't want to be depressed by the reality of his limitations. I wanted him to stay perfect. My hero. He was my first love. The other lovers had been skirmishes really, a lot of them, but fleeting – occasionally stimulating, often anonymous, sometimes in Wyoming. I had experienced excitement, and orgasms, mostly external, some internal, and I had very occasionally discovered something new, but I had never had a long-term relationship, or any real knowledge of men beyond their sexual needs, their tastes in pop music and the ideas they had picked up at art school. I was fascinated and mystified by them but I didn't trust them. I would look at them in the same way one stares at big-toothed mammals in the zoo, but with less respect due to the fact that I had studied history.

I didn't care if men liked me or fancied me, and this isolated me from many other women, as that was all they thought about – being desired, wanted, whatever. I watched as they twisted themselves to conform with perceived notions of femininity, losing themselves in the process, then wondering why it wasn't working. I was aware of my soul, aware of authenticity, and naïve about the challenges of non-conformism. I didn't realise at that time that to do as you pleased, to wear what you wanted, to relish independence, to savour self-containment – these things were unusual and they would take courage to sustain.

I was seen as eccentric, possibly unmanageable, but sexy enough to make the effort worthwhile. Some men were drawn to me, enjoying the challenge; others hated me on sight. They knew I would never pander to their egos. I would always disagree with them if I felt like it; I would go to Budapest if I felt like it. It took a daddy to reign me in, a man who knew the script without having read it. I didn't appreciate Daddy as he deserved during the time that I knew him because I thought there were many daddies around the place, that the world was full of middle-aged men yearning for manqué pubescents. I was right to a certain extent, but most men were confined. They could not pursue their desires, prohibited, as they were, by morality or marriage or both. I did not realise that Daddy was unique and that I was lucky to have found him.

Was he scared? Is that why he had to have control? The answer: perhaps. But he wasn't scared of me, either as a personality or as a representative of the gender. His first and only wife had died in a car crash when they were in their twenties. He was scared of chaos. He was scared of the fates over which he had no power, and, not having any faith, religious or otherwise, he was alone in his fear.

If a lampshade was out of place he suffered until it was replaced and by replacing it he calmed his nerves. If I was late he became anxious, but covered it up with his designated guardian role. He did not have children but he did have love. It had to go somewhere. I like to think that he was a generous man who was genuinely interested in creating pleasure.

I, meanwhile, was a visitor in his life and a guest in his houses. I liked the formality – it was distant and it was erotic and it meant that I was attended to. As a guest I received the privileges required by good manners. As a child bride I would have become a wife and then part of the furniture. I would probably have had to engage in interminable discussions about how the Aubusson should be upholstered or restored.

He did ask me once if I wanted children. I told him no and I wasn't kidding.

'Do you?' I said nervously.

'I did once, when I was married, but I think it was because I wanted to please my wife. Occasionally I wonder who I'm going to leave everything to, who deserves it, how alone I will be in the end, what my contribution has been. But, strangely, I didn't want to be a father – I didn't want to have to deal with the crying and whining and fighting and school fees and the worry and disappointment of it all. Parenthood seems a very thankless task to me. But there's a part of me, well . . .'

'You can leave everything to me if you like,' I mentioned.

'Ah, Stella. First of all you haven't sucked up to me nearly enough. Secondly, you won't be here at the end. I will have a young nurse and she will get it all.'

'Hey!'

My heart lurched with this prophecy. I didn't like the idea of not being there, not having a daddy, my daddy. Perhaps I should marry the bloody man, I thought to myself, if only to stop nurses predating him. It wouldn't be the end of the world. I could probably do what I liked to a certain extent.

I had heard that it was unwise to marry for sex, but I would have liked to be engaged in a camp 1950s kind of way, with a blinding diamond on the finger and a dress with a skirt large enough to offer shelter to three homeless people. My grandmother wore one of those vast gowns when she came out at Queen Charlotte's Ball. 'Darling, what a night! The whole room wanted to marry me.' By marrying, of course, she meant sex, which was the same thing in her day. She certainly could not have had sex before marriage because the clothes took three hours to remove by which time the man had died of exhaustion.

An engagement would be a novelty. I could enjoy it as an improvised performance piece designed to entertain. I didn't genuinely want to commit to Daddy or any thing for that matter. If I found myself with a geranium the responsibility began to worry me. They always died.

I was aware, at some level, of the unromantic truth that our love affair would end. I did not worry about this. The sex was spectacular and absorbing and enough. We were distant but close. Our world was safe and sexual and imbued with complete trust and perfect understanding, for which honesty was demanded and this was not always easy.

I don't like cunnilingus. I just don't. Some might say this makes me a bad lover, but what is a bad lover? Daddy never asked me if I thought he was a good lover or a bad lover. If he had, I would have wondered if the question was based on a desire to know or a need for affirmation. Some people think there are no good or bad lovers because it is all about love and chemistry. They are wrong. There is such a thing as skill; there is such a thing as experience and generosity and this can turn someone into a very good fuck.

Having said that, just as I did not care if people thought I was boring or not, I did not care whether they thought I was a good lover or not. I didn't really care what people thought of me, in general, as there were very few individuals whose judgement I respected. If I had walked into a room and heard my lover say, 'Big bush and boring in bed' I would have dismissed this as a reflection on the speaker rather than on me. I had confidence in my own act. I was lucky in that. I would rather provoke horror or mystification than gormless appraisals based on ignorance and the need to undermine. Having said that, there were some things about sex that I had problems with when I met Daddy.

I do not like cunnilingus. I would rather have anal sex in the street; I would rather be chained to a wall and possessed; I would rather do a lap dance; I would rather be pissed on. I like to think my mind is open – open to scenarios, as limitless as the imagination, but I do not like their tongues down there, like annoying lapdogs. Was that what Pekingese were bred for? I have often wondered.

I cannot indulge the male delusion that their tongues are possessed with miraculous powers. I am neither that kind nor that dishonest. But Daddy enjoyed cunnilingus and I fought it. I fought him off, pushed him away, but he thought it was part of fight and foreplay and simply used it to overcome me. I fought him more. In the end he tied me up to do it. He would tie me to his four-poster bed, ankles at each end, legs spread out and wide, lips and clit exposed. He would gag me so that I could scream all I wanted and neither he nor the Borough of Kensington and Chelsea would have to hear it. The gagging allowed me to surrender and God knows I needed the help. But I was not screaming because I was coming, I was screaming with frustration and fear. Presented with permission to submit, I screamed the scream of a woman who did not wish the man to have control over her body, let alone the sheer exposure of orgasmic release.

If I wriggled out of his way, trying to avoid that torturing tongue which tickled and lapped with relentless intensity and horrifying intimacy, he would slap me hard on the top of the thigh, so the pain started to meld with the tongue and everything tingled and melted.

Slapping, kissing and then the licking of the clit – it was agony. I wanted to kill him, but on he would go, and I knew he would not stop until I came, so I had to come, I had to let go and eventually, after a lot of fighting and shouting and thoughts of revenge, my psyche heaved itself into surrender and I came, noisy and cross but compliant. Some men would have thought all this was an effort just to lick a girl's fanny, but Daddy liked it. He liked winning.

I was more compliant around fellatio and sucked his dick when and where he told me to. I liked his dick. It was big and clean and circumcised and it fitted beautifully into my mouth. I liked to do as he instructed and, by so doing, perfect the craft on his behalf – designing my technique so that it suited him. I didn't care about anybody else at that point.

In general I did as I was told sexually, and conformed to his desires. If he wanted a blow job he got it. I loved him and I complied. I didn't always like giving blow jobs to men, and I did not like the way they so rudely expected the woman to delight in the presentation of the penis for consumption. I can only assume that men thought that women would be pleased to see their sexual organs because men themselves like to see those of women. But it doesn't work like that. Just because men delight in any old cunt, as long as it's up close and personal, women are far more discriminating. The vibrant helmet and shiny head has to be attached to something vaguely acceptable.

I sucked him in the way that he wanted to be sucked, which was to take the top into my mouth, suck quite hard, massage him with my tongue, while gently fondling the shaft and stroking the balls. His dick was both wide and long, and, erect, would never have gone down my throat without causing crying and gagging, which is hardly erotic or comfortable. I wasn't a giraffe after all. But the beginning was fun, the head growing larger in my mouth, the power as my tongue flicked against it, his pleasure as the blood surged through and he struggled to keep the physical and mental control – he exercised to maintain both, allowing himself slowly to orgasm, and controlling me as he controlled himself.

His generosity to my needs was boundless so he taught me how to give. I had been selfish up to that point because I had mostly encountered selfishness. And ineptitude. Having said that, the first time he came in my mouth I was both surprised and furious. I spat the spunk straight back in his face. He smiled and wiped the gob off his cheek with great dignity. He was about to say something, when I got up and stalked out of the room. He found me stiff with anger in the master bathroom, wrapped in a big white towel and smoking a forbidden cigarette. I didn't know why I hated him I just did. My mouth was set in a brat pout and I was actually shaking.

'What's the problem?' he asked.

'Fuck off.'

'Don't speak to me like that.'

I pouted and was subsumed by wordless teenage rage.

'Stella, stop being silly. You tell your Daddy everything, you know that.' He took the cigarette out of my mouth, flushed it under the tap and put it in the bin. 'Stella!'

I breathed out, braced myself and spoke the truth. 'I don't like come,' I said. 'I just don't. I don't like the way you're supposed to like it in your face, all over your body, oozing out of every orifice like porno. I can't understand why they – those film people – expect the world to respect their semen and I can't understand why they make women drink it. I can't worship a fluid just because it is full of male chromosomes. Why are they so proud of their jism when they've all got it, and the ability to produce it, and godawful abundance is a mundane commonality? I mean I can worship courage, and originality of perspective, and charm, and a sense of humour, but I don't like that white stuff and I can't pretend to. It makes me feel sick. I don't want it in my eyes or mouth or ears for that matter.'

He smiled. 'I have not come across this particular revulsion before – or no woman has admitted to it anyway. I'm afraid I had not thought about whether you would mind or not; I guess I assumed that you wouldn't. As I like your fluids, as you describe them, I assumed you would have no objection to mine. Furthermore we have established that I do not ask permission for things. You do as you're told.'

'There are limits.'

'You're right. There are limits and so there should be. We should have talked about it. We should talk about every-thing that we do, especially when we play like we do. There's a lot of room for mistakes and hurt. There are things I don't like to do as well. I have no intention of licking your arsehole, for instance. Though I have every intention of putting both my fingers and dick into it. Now come here.'

He kissed me. I kissed him back. The towel dropped and he hugged me and sucked my breasts. Then he ran a bath and put me in it. He washed my hair. He massaged my neck and back. He spoke to me softly as one speaks softly to a child who needs encouragement. 'I am going to shave you tomorrow,' he said, 'and I am going to study your naughty little cunt.'

My anger melted away but I never knew its source. I still don't. Daddy always knew what to do and he always made me feel better and quite often helped me move away from my unhelpful beliefs and secret little anxieties. He looked like a straight person from Chelsea, but he had a realm of understanding that was way beyond mine. He was not shocked by anything except bad manners. He was extraordinary.

I liked driving with Daddy. He had a dark-green Merc and he drove beautifully, with confidence and skill. He always clicked my seat belt for me. At the end of the journey, he would get out, open the door for me, unlock the seat belt and take my hand to help me. He would always kiss me on the lips no matter what had happened on the journey, and things always did happen, inevitably, as we couldn't be together for more than half an hour without winding each other up.

I tended to initiate the dramas. I was provocative, proactive and younger. He had less energy and, being male, might have focused on the navigation and driving rather than on me. His stance was to ensure that there was a ruler and a hairbrush in the glove compartment in the event that either were needed. I threw them out the window once, which didn't do me any good. He had a crop in the boot, so he bent me over the bonnet of the car, and striped my buttocks and thighs until my shrieks frightened the birds out of the trees. I couldn't sit down for a week.

So driving was fun.

He often gave me lectures about my behaviour. 'You're a naughty girl and I'm going to send you away.'

'I don't want to go away unless it's to look at birds in Madagascar.'

'I can't imagine what your reports would be like. It would be a waste of money trying to educate you.'

'I don't need to be educated, thank you very much. I have a 2.1 degree in English literature.'

I would become irritated, or wet, or both, and then have to beg for permission to play with myself, stilettos up on the dashboard, legs akimbo, rubbing myself while he tried to concentrate on the road and grew hard.

On one of these occasions, he accused me of being immature and selfish. He said the point of sexual subjugation was not merely to cause pleasure in the moment, but to lead to a place where insights and useful changes could be made. The point of subjugation, he said, apart from the obvious catharsis of physical release and the sensuality of abnegation, was to learn about humility and, through that subtle realisation, achieve the transcendence of unconditional generosity.

I needed to learn about compromise. To accept the defects of a lover or friend was to learn about the hate in love. If I walked away from my own sun, he said, I would discover interesting aspects about myself and they would lead me to give more of myself to others. In his opinion this was the only way to achieve and maintain personal equilibrium.

I looked out of the window so he couldn't see that I was rolling my eyes. It was as if Sid Vicious had never lived. I had never put myself out for anybody and did not intend to start just because he suggested it. I did love him in my own way, but I had not been tested. My inner life, self-involved to the point of autism, was engaged in the pursuit of pleasure and the deflection of ennui.

Unconditional love indeed. There was no such thing. Any honest altruist would admit that their pursuit assuaged their personal feelings of worthlessness. Mother love was a simple evolvement to protect the gene. When I was living on the lower East Side, I wrote 'Kill all hippies' in my own blood on the wall of my apartment. There was a reason for this. I did actually believe that the 1960s produced a generation of drug-addled defectives whose legacy was a lesson in how to be ineffectual. Love chaos. Hate Ashbury. Never trust a flower. Especially snowdrops with their silly meek heads telling lies about the end of winter. So I told him he was talking hippy shit.

He screeched the car to a halt in the middle of a country lane and parked it down a muddy track. Then he dragged me out of the passenger seat. It was summer. I was wearing a black miniskirt, a crumpled vintage blouse, which I had ripped the sleeves off so it was like a waistcoat, and pair of idiotically high burgundy velvet court shoes, with five-inch clumpy heels, a round toe and a tiny platform on the sole.

There had been rain so there was mud. I wondered afterwards if Daddy knew the place, deep in the country-side, isolated, with fields and stiles and on the edge of a wood. He dragged me through a dark-green tunnel made of overgrown hazel and beech trees. His own immaculate grey trousers and shiny shiny black brogues gathered mud and leaves as he gripped my wrist and led me, tottering and grumbling, further into the woods.

There were actual puddles and soft mud so that it was genuinely difficult to walk. I whined about the shoes being ruined and it was his fault and he would have to buy me some more, as they became dark with filth and the mud started to cake up my bare legs almost to my knees.

He did not acknowledge either my voice or my presence.

We walked for hours. Later he said it was ten minutes max and I was exaggerating as usual. But it seemed like hours with the mud and nettles and briars pricking the legs.

'Fuck you,' I observed. 'Why am I being punished? Because I called you a hippy? Or because I dare to contradict you?'

I had not to that date met a man who could bear being contradicted by a woman.

'Neither. Firstly, I was never a hippy. I lived in Geneva for most of the sixties. Secondly, I don't consider it to be the insult that you intended. You're going to learn what I mean. You're going to learn the pleasure of giving yourself to me.'

He picked up sticks, tossed them away, picked them up again, found what he wanted.

'I want to pee.'

'You'll have to wait.'

'I want to pee.'

'Oh for God's sake. Give me your pants and squat down there in front of me.'

'It's a bit difficult with these shoes and the mud,' I pointed out.

'Get on with it, Stella, I'm losing my patience.'

I held his shoulder and he pulled my pants down for me, struggling to get them off my ankles and over the clumpy shoes. I crouched down and peed on his shiny shiny Church's brogues.

Seeing what I had done, which, by the way, was not on purpose, he shoved my knickers into my mouth, pushed me onto all fours in the leaves and mud, hoiked my arse towards him and whipped me like a dog with the stick.

And I yelped like a dog. 'Ow! No!'

He whipped my bare behind with that flicky bit of willow so hard I thought it would break. But it didn't, he just went on and on, whipping me so that I could feel every stripe slash into my white flesh. I thought he would never stop. My face was down in the dirt, I smelled the earth and felt the pain, the warm excitement on my clitoris. There was only the noise of the stick on my arse, the coo of a lone pigeon and Daddy's breathing, as he concentrated on the pleasure of his power, the slick skilful punishment, his erection, the silent place of mutual sexuality, the ultimate trust as peculiarity is faced and enjoyed in a place of great pain where nobody is hurt.

He waited. Silence. I connected with the flaming pain seeping across my buttocks and thighs. I could feel the blood pumping to the wounded places. The endorphins kicked in. I entered the zone of the submissive: spaced out, compliant, smiling. The pain brought me into the present, as in the present as it was possible to be. There was only the moment. The mulch. The smell of Daddy and earth. Thoughts disappeared. The mind rested. I thought he had finished with me and I started to relax, but no. I was for it this time. He whipped me again, stick striping flesh, on and on.

Overcome, I burst into tears.

He stopped. Put his hand up my cunt to make sure I was wet. He took the pants out of my mouth and put them in his pocket. Then he pulled me up into a standing positon, put his hand on my chin and lifted my tear-stained red face towards him. I stopped sobbing and calmed down. He kissed me and said firmly, but gently, 'You will listen to me when I am speaking to you.'

I gave him my filthy hand and he led me back to the car. He helped me into the passenger seat and I sat there with my hot arse bare against the upholstery, my thighs separated to show him my throbbing swollen lips. He did my seat belt up and said, 'Now calm down.'

My hands were resting on the seat but, as he looked down at me, my mons convulsed and I came spontaneously. He watched. I came again. He smiled and the corners of his eyes crinkled. I was completely in love with him and he was right. At that moment I would have done anything for him.

Daddy owned a house in the country. Its origins were Elizabethan but it had fallen down and been built again many times so that one aspect was timbered and another was Queen Anne. It had no symmetry, but it did have character, as with the years additions had been made reflecting the taste, ego and budget of the various owners. Now it had turrets and chimneys, arches and a courtyard, and gardens which required the attention of three men. There were stables and a swimming pool, various walled gardens and woods, and, in the distance, 500 acres of Sussex.

A round tower dominated one corner. Ivy grew up it and it had windows all around so that you could see for miles over the countryside. That was my bedroom. I could stare out at 360 degrees of fields and forests, cows and sheep, and overgrown lanes going nowhere.

It had once been used for guests, but Daddy adapted it for me. I slept in a four-poster bed with heavy cream silk drapes and hooks banged into each post at various levels. There was a polished walnut bookshelf, a table, a green sofa, a fireplace, an ottoman chest and a large white wardrobe. The bathroom was perfect, with a Victorian bath and mirrors, and a comprehensive selection of oils and creams. Daddy was keen on a bath product. He was never out of the shops in Jermyn Street, sniffing around and making selections. I was always well oiled and scented. Not that I needed creams, except when he had me on all fours and was easing himself into my rectum, easing his hard shaft up me with his big hands playing over my lips and clit, bringing me to climax as he ejaculated into me. He would bring me to an orgasm with his hands and then wrap me in a huge white cotton towelling bathrobe.

My 'apartment' was accessed by a winding stone staircase, which was difficult to climb in high heels. Daddy would follow me as I struggled up, handbag, gloves, coat, seamed stockings, leopard-skin ankle boots with needle heels. He would laugh as I made my ungraceful climb, and enjoy an erection at the sight of my struggle. A woman compromised always aroused him. 'I don't know why really,' he once tried to explain. 'But I suspect the truth is that there is an atavistic sensibility that knows a girl compromised by a high heel is a girl that cannot run away. And a girl in high heels carrying things in her hands is a girl that can be taken.'

He did like to rape me. Though rape, of course, is the wrong word, meaning, as it still does, an illegal lack of consent. Perhaps one of these days the tiny circles of tired feminist academia will stop fighting with itself and arrive at a pertinent word for consensual rape – a word that denotes the mastery over a fantasy and the realisation of a set of circumstances that do not involve a hideous sex criminal, but a handsome man following one down the street and into an alley. His dick is clean, he is neither obese nor putrescent nor what the neighbours call a 'loner'. He rips your clothes off because you want him to. You bite and scratch. He holds you down. Rape. But not.

I knew when he wanted to rape me, because he would tell me to go somewhere and he would meet me later. He would say, 'Stella, go and get some lettuces from the vegetable garden, I will meet you up there. I've got some calls to make. I've laid your outfit on your bed. Go on now.'

There was always a 'rape' costume, which added to the delight and which was always ripped to shreds so it was a new one every time. Outfits to get raped in? Blimey. The queens in Paris have created many styles of apparel in which to be violated. Daddy chose carefully. Sometimes he bought things specially. Sometimes he selected from the clothes hanging on immaculate wooden hangers in my white wardrobe. He chose perfect hangers, though he never beat me with one. Not enough give, he said. And I agreed. He preferred a whippy willow switch.

I learned to be quite tidy for him, which was not my natural bent. If he came to the bedroom and found clothes on the floor, he would slap me until I screamed out loud, or sobbed, or both. And though this was very enjoyable, and I often did it on purpose, I also began to appreciate a sense of order. I found it relaxing to fold and hang and arrange. I agreed with him that it was spoiled not to appreciate the things that he had bought for me, and slutty to leave them around in filthy piles for Susan to pick up.

'It's getting dark,' I might say. 'I won't be able to see anything.'

'Take a torch.'

I would walk into the lowering dusk of the summer's evening, an innocent shepherdess entering an Arcadia of dangerous swains. The growing darkness and the knowledge that I was to be leaped upon and taken by force always made my heart beat, the more so as the minutes went on, and he always let me wander for at least fifteen minutes – and fifteen minutes can be a long time when your heart is beating and the shadows are growing around the trees, the shrubs, the gates, the outhouses, and all the time you are listening for the crunch of the footstep on gravel, or heavy breathing, or a fleeting shadow behind the statue of Samson slaying the Philistine.

Daddy was good at creeping. He might have had ninja training. He was so dark and silent. He always surprised me, no matter how alert I was, how aware of the so-called danger of this arrival. I would pad around nervously in the darkening gardens, the shadows of the vines creeping fingers up the grey stone walls, my hair prickling on my head, the old cells performing their evolutionary purpose by trying to make me look bigger in the face of danger. The danger wasn't real, of course, but as when watching the scene of a thriller, the mind and body lost a sense of the present and reacted to the pretence. He usually grabbed me from behind, and I would shriek out loud from genuine shock and seconds of actual fear. He would put a leather-gloved hand over my mouth, though this would not stop the screaming. Then he would push me over onto the ground, sit on top of me and simply rip my clothes off. The little lace blouse, the balcony bra, the sweet summer skirt, which had done no harm to anyone, except, perhaps, reveal the round orbs of my arse to anyone lucky enough to be walking behind me. Whatever it was, he tore it off, so that my breasts, hard as nails, were his to suck and gobble and bite. My pants would be torn off as well. Literally ripped. Which only a determined and strong man could do, as it is not as easy as it looks, unless the knickers are very flimsy, which they usually were.

I would fight like hell. Well. Who wouldn't? I would punch and scream and kick, and use all my strength against this brute force, but he overwhelmed me by the simple fact of being stronger than me. I liked to feel his strength. There was some part of me that did not want to win. I wanted to know his force was overwhelming, that I could not fight it. But I would fight. I like fighting. I would try to push him away with every muscle in my body, but he would sit on me and pull my face towards his with his hands. I was forced to receive his tongue. One hand would push my arms behind my head and the other would go into me, his fingers penetrating into the wetness between my kicking legs. Finally, he would flip me over, take his cock out of his flies and simply fuck me while I was still pretending I didn't want him to and he was a bastard.

He would tell me I got everything I asked for. Which was true, of course. He would come inside me, stand up, put his dick back into his trousers and walk off into the night, leaving me spread and filthy and alone in the dark. Dazed and dirty, in a post-coital, post-orgasm state of confusion. I would then walk back to the house, looking like a crime scene – filthy face, ripped clothes, but with a wet throbbing cunt and the happiness that arrives from a good seeing-to. He always kissed me when I returned. We had been in a strange place after all. If we had remained distant in that intense moment, I might have gone into some supernormal victimhood, which would have been unhealthy and unfair.

It was important to reconnect immediately. We would sit cosy in the small sitting room. He would have a glass of red wine and I would have a glass of Coca Cola and a dirty face. Daddy would smile and stroke my hair and ask me if I had enjoyed myself.

On the other hand, I could spend two days in the country and receive no attention at all. Daddy would go out somewhere and Jimmy would tell me that he had left instructions that I wasn't allowed any of the car keys, but I could take the dogs for a walk if I wanted. By the time I heard the car on the drive, I was sulky and resentful. On one occasion, I heard him stomping around trying to find me. I hid behind one of the tapestries in the corridor, like Polonius.

'Come out at once. What do you think you're doing?'
Hiding.

* * *

I spent the whole of August 1985 with Daddy in the country but I was never allowed to stay the night in the master bedroom. I visited in the evenings and in the mornings, when summoned. Daddy did not allow me to share his 'quarters' – we had separate territories as in Victorian gothic novels. He slept very badly, he said, and worse if there was someone hot and breathing beside him.

'And you snore,' I pointed out.

'I do not snore.'

'You do snore. I've just had a complaint from a man living in Inverness. He said he heard you. He said it was noise pollution.'

'Don't be absurd.'

Anyway, we slept in different bedrooms and I didn't mind as he did snore. I always slept very well, which he found profoundly irritating. He took great delight in climbing up the stairs at 4 a.m., if he was having a bad night, and simply entering me while I was asleep, so I woke up to find his big dick inside me and his breath on the back of my neck.

Once I knocked on his bedroom door in the middle of the night. I pretended I had had a nightmare, but actually I just wanted to have sex. He was awake. He was always awake. He was wearing only pyjama bottoms, striped, from Brooks Brothers. He bought them in bulk when he went to New York. He took me by the hand, led me past the portraits and back up to my room, staying with me until I went back to sleep.

'I want a glass of water.'

'I don't want to hear another word out of you.'

'I want sex.'

I put my own fingers into my cunt and showed him how wet I was.

But he just smiled. 'Wank yourself off. You know I like to watch you.'

I rubbed myself. He then stood over me, watching, tall and stern, looking down. 'Go on. I want to see you come.'

So I rubbed until I came and when I did he put his three fingers up me and manipulated me from a small orgasm into waves of pleasure and until I lost myself.

'Now go to sleep. I'm very tired.' He licked the juice off my fingers then kissed me on the lips. He turned the light out, but left the one on in the corridor. I heard his footsteps walk further and further away, and I thought about him as I fell to sleep.

What more could a girl want?

If he came to my room and I wasn't there, there would be trouble as I had to tell him if I was going out. He always needed to know exactly where I was. If I wasn't where I was expected to be, he would find me and punish me. Once he was looking for me and I was in the garden and he simply picked me up and carried me into the house, pulled me over his knee on a chair in the hall, pulled down my pants and spanked me in the hall where there was a risk of any member of the staff walking through. Then I had to stand in the corner, if you please, face to the wall, skirt and pants in a pool on the floor, with flaming buttocks and a stag's head staring down at me.

'You will stay there until tea time,' he said.

He had to know where I was.

Another day I took the Ferrari and rammed it at 100 miles an hour around the estate and one of the tenants complained. Daddy was waiting for me when I screeched it up the drive and did a handbrake turn as I had been taught by a Harrovian in 1973 (his parents had been away at the time). It was Daddy's fault for both owning a Ferrari and leaving the keys in it. Actually it was Jimmy's fault, and I think he got told off for it, unless he did it on purpose because he was bored and wanted to see what would happen.

Daddy was waiting for me, all gothic stepfather, in the hall.

'Give me the keys and go to your room at once.'

I had to wait in my weird tower for a day, thinking about what was going to happen to me, masturbating at the thought of his fury, regretting that my days of speed were over.

He came up at about 5 p.m. and tied me up. I was lying on my back, my ankles attached by silk to the hook on each pole of the bed; there were four hooks at different levels. This time he tied my ankles quite high up so that my cunt was raised up and open. My arms were tied to the remaining poles.

I wanted to pee, but he didn't return so I had no relief. In the end I just went, on the sheets and everything. Fifteen minutes later he found me in a stain of wet, untied me, and put me over his knee for a hard slippering.

Sometimes he came to my room and read to me and then left again and it turned me on so much I couldn't sleep for wanting to fuck him.

I always had breakfast with him, in the dining room, eggs in silver tureens on a warming plate at one end of the room, newspapers. I was expected to wear long white nighties with puff sleeves and pie-crust frills or baby-doll pyjamas. He bought them for me in the teen sections of smart department stores. He had a Harrods card, as I recall, which I found fascinating. My only experience of Harrods being that it was an easy place from which to shoplift.

He would sit at the head of the table and I would sit next to him in my dressing gown, very demure, drinking my orange juice and attempting to behave myself. Immature for my age? Probably. Who knows what you're supposed to be like when you're 25? I was inclined to avoid responsibility and pursue pleasure and I was encouraged to do so by

Daddy. I did not have to work and did not wish to. I did not want a career. I did not want a baby. I did not aspire to the usual fulfilments. I aspired to the fulfilment of fantasy and it was a full-time job, exploring its possibilities and tuning into its adventure. I did not feel stunted or weird or atrophied. I felt free.

It suited us both to play, though neither of us thought much of the consequences. I certainly didn't, but I rarely thought of the consequences of anything. I had taken all the drugs handed to me without any thought at all except for the effects on the present and I would take any sado-masochistic scenario with the same pathological panache. It was lucky for me that Daddy was more restrained. They were cutting each other in the clubs, cutting and using cow prods and lashing and fisting. It was all going on. We were innocents in comparison, though sophisticated in terms of head games, or psycho-sexual drama as it has since become known.

Daddy liked me to be young. He didn't want an adult. He loved me in this fixed place where there was wildness and hope and he could exercise convincing control. The closer we became the more controlling he became and I realised how neurotic he was – that there was fear there. I occasionally saw glimpses of it, in the worry, or fleeting panic if Jimmy was two minutes late, or I had taken an umbrella from the stand and not put it back, or there was a smear on his silver.

He needed me to be in my place and he was moulding me to the image that he wanted as surely as a sculptor moulded clay. He knew that on some level I needed him and that was essential for him as it protected him against his own fears that I would leave him. We both started to become the people that we had created for each other. I didn't bother with my old self; I hardly knew who it was any more.

I became less interested in or involved with the world that I had lived in before I met him. The old schoolfriends; the Manhattan bohos and Chelsea queens. I was his naughty Stella, wayward ward who would do anything and stay adolescent, sometimes younger if we felt like it.

I was protected from reality by the sun of the summer days and the boundaries of the estate but, occasionally, travelling into the local town to shop, I found myself being his creation without making any conscious effort to walk into it. It was as if the part had taken over the actress and when she walked off set she was still the sixteen year old that needed to be taken in hand, dependent on the authority against which she rebelled, in love with his protection and control.

I didn't make any effort to choose for myself any more because Daddy automatically made all decisions for me at the same time that he made them for himself. I ate what he told me to, wore what he told me to, spent my days pretty much as he told me to. I didn't mind. I liked it. I liked being at one with him and losing myself entirely; I lost the burden of the committee in the head, which had previously asked inconvenient questions about the meaning of the void and where I thought I was going and did I actually care about anything and wouldn't it be nice to be dead, or at least on a long holiday during which one was unconscious.

I had sex with him whenever he desired it so I was in a constant state of sexual arousal, which made me agitated and obsessed with having him in me. The hours were filled with his hands and his skin and his cock and his warmth. We were connected. Slowly, as the summer days went by, I hardly noticed that I was leaving some aspects of my personality behind and turning into his creation. I did not even notice when Daddy took me by the hand and led me into the local hairdresser. My hair, now long and black, had become wild in the country, receiving no attention and only occasionally wearing a hairband because Daddy made me, and being brushed because Daddy brushed it. I wouldn't have dreamed of doing so myself.

Daddy asked the woman give me a Louise Brooks bob with a very short psycho fringe. He turned me back into the mad urchin with whom he liked to play.

There were some days, however, that the rebel returned from wherever she had been hiding and reclaimed her rights. The old Stella drew her bow and aimed her arrows and walked away, unmoved and unafraid.

Towards the end of August, I spent most of my time by the swimming pool. The days were hot and the pool was gorgeous, heated and azure and clear. It was surrounded by walls covered in sweet-smelling creepers around which butterflies and bees hovered.

The pool house was a listed art deco building. There were pink arches and statues of deco women in swimming costumes. All the mosaics and paving stones were original. There were also changing rooms and a bar with a sound system and fluffy cotton towels in eau de Nil. It was perfect.

I am always happy next to water and in it. I spent hours up there playing The Cult and The Cure and the Batcave mob as loudly as possible on the sound system. I would have smoked cigarettes and drunk the champagne in the fridge but I didn't dare. Daddy would have smelled them on my breath and sent me back to the house, or worse. And I didn't want to sit in my bedroom, bored, looking out at the sunny day and waiting for a whipping.

Daddy had bought me a soft white bathrobe for poolside lounging. He approved of me sitting by the pool because it meant he knew where I was. He didn't allow me to wear a top, as he liked my breasts to be brown, which they soon were. I had various teeny bikini bottoms, which showed half my buttocks from the back and the fact that he had shaved my bush from the front. One, my favourite, was white cotton and made by Norma Kamali. It looked better and better as the sun tanned my skin and my legs grew browner by the day. He demanded that my toenails were always perfectly painted and sometimes underwent this task himself, giving me an immaculate pedicure. He loved my feet and would kiss them. The heat made us both soft and receptive and up for even more activity than usual.

Daddy didn't like The Cult or The Cure and thoroughly resented their representation in his environment, but I liked to dance semi-naked to 'The Lovecats' and that was all there was to it.

One hot afternoon I was sunbathing, comfortable and warm, reading a *Jackie* annual from behind my Ray-Bans and listening to the Sisters of Mercy. Daddy turned up to swim, as was his habit, at about 3 p.m. He was wearing khaki chinos and a short-sleeved white cotton shirt and dark glasses with brown lenses and tortoise-shell frames. He was gaunt and glamorous; he could have been in a Rat Pack film, not at all out of place. I looked at his mouth and loved it as always. If you love the mouth you love the man, though I suppose it does slightly depend on what comes out of it.

This particular weekend was a bank holiday and the end of the summer was drawing near. I dreaded it. I did not want to leave my daddy and go back to horrible London and face the winter.

'Turn that music off, Stella, please.'

I remained as stationary as it is possible to be without actually having rigor mortis. 'Amphetamine Logic' was on quite loud so it was easy to pretend I hadn't heard him.

He came up and pulled my foot so that I lost my balance and the book fell onto the paving stones.

'Hey!'

'Do as you are told.'

'Don't be so horrible. I hate you.'

'If you're rude you'll go to your room.'

'Fuck off.'

'Do as you're told! You will learn some manners and you will learn to respect me.'

'What's to respect?'

I wasn't in the greatest of moods. Feeling gloomy and irritable, I was ready to hurt him. I looked up at him eyeless through the shades and returned to the book with an insouciance which I knew would drive him mad.

He flinched. I knew that my last remark had touched a nerve where low self-esteem melded with the money issues that inevitably arrive with inherited wealth, a status that is undeserved and unfair. Daddy did not rate his achievements very highly. He knew that, in the end, he was a rich businessman with private means that he had not earned and that he was of little use to anybody except himself. He did not have much to be proud of, never having been challenged by any of the things that life tends to throw at people. He had not done much. And he certainly had done little that was good.

Where was his mark? He had no children, no immortal legacy. He owned twenty occasional tables and some uninteresting paintings. When he went he would go and few people would notice or care. When I asked what there was to respect, his dark part knew that I was right; even when I did enact respect it was the result of our sophisticated foreplay rather than from honest appraisal.

He went silent and cold and without a word took out his dick and pissed on me. I didn't realise what he was doing until it was too late and I was well and truly covered, all over my stomach, my breasts, my thighs.

Leaping to my feet, I spat in his face. He slapped me on the cheek, not hard, but it stung and brought tears to my eyes. I pushed him out of the way, stomped to the pool and dived in. I had not swum half a length away from him when I felt him on top of me, naked, his dick hard and wet pressing against my legs. He pulled down my bikini pants, and manhandled me back to the shallow end. I struggled but I knew I was not going to win. He was like an octopus all over me, arms and legs, overwhelming my wet body.

Pushing me down on the shallow step where the water was about five inches, he stood over me naked, his stomach and legs firm and brown, his erection rock hard.

'Stay there,' he shouted. 'Don't you dare move.'

Some men tie up their 'slaves' in order to retain the control that they need. Daddy did tie me up sometimes, but it was rarely necessary. His personality was enough; his voice and his strength. He rarely shouted and, slightly frightened, I lay naked in the water watching him – a tall brown naked man with wet hair smoothed over a lupine forehead. My shaved labia poked up from the blue water, smooth and pink and without innocence. He looked down and smiled. Then he began to masturbate, slowly at first, with cruel crude self-indulgent movements, hand down shaft, just him and his dick and a bad ladygirl object sprawled below him. Could I have been anybody? Did it matter that it was me? Did he know it was me or had the brain surrendered to the pleasure principles, the compulsions of orgasm?

He pummelled his shaft until he came all over me in great gobs of porno gunk, on my tits, stomach, thighs, lips.

Satisfied, he turned his back on me, dived back into the pool, hoiked himself out of the deep end and walked naked to the house without looking back.

I lay there, breathing hard, his come all over me, the waves from his dive lapping onto my legs. I put my hand into myself, and kept it there as the sun dried his white juice into my skin and I began to smell of almonds and salt.

6. 1985–6

I had been seeing Daddy for three years before discovering that he was bisexual. It was a shock at first, though with hindsight I should have guessed. It wasn't that he was keeping it from me, more that we were involved with each other and other options had not been discussed. Then one of his male lovers turned up with a cheap suitcase and the world went dark. I wanted my daddy to myself, but here was this youth: handsome and needy, the brother that I had never had and did not want competing for the father I had never had and did want.

We were introduced in the drawing room at Cheyne Walk. 'Stella, Mandy; Mandy, Stella.'

So he was called Mandy before you had even started.

I remember I had a lot of eyeliner on that evening and the most wonderful vintage Quant minidress. They didn't help.

I'm not often speechless but I gazed upon this arriviste without a word. He was small, brown and shiny. His sleeveless Lycra singlet was orange, and he was wearing a hairband in his shoulder-length black hair. His jeans had been carefully ripped and, at the crotch, the denim had stretched and whitened from the pressure of attempting to contain him. His aftershave was enough to make a cow fall over. His face, in repose, was female and petulant, but the smile was radiant and childlike. I could see that Mandy was possessed of the kind of charm that can be turned into a skill, but I wanted to punch him in the face.

He was from Venezuela.

He could salsa.

He was hell.

Mandy and I eyed each other up while Daddy failed to notice anything except the new boy. It was as if I wasn't in the room. I was invisible to the human eye.

'What's Caracas like?' I said.

'A sheetole,' Mandy replied.

He had clear cold brown eyes, which promised savage fury. I had seen this expression on the faces of other queens and knew that if they decided to blow, they blew. There was a hag on my grandmother's estate who used to talk about energies and power and magic, and she always said, 'You have powers, dear, use them carefully.' She said to use beer on your hair as well, which is a bad idea, and I should have guessed from looking at hers, which was thin and mousy and stood up on her head when it was about to thunder. The combination of my childhood solitude and her haggish advice about the content of the invisible honed my awareness about things like coincidence and atmosphere and sexual effect. I had an acute sense of danger and a healthy distrust. These things came to my aid at this moment.

I soon realised Mandy was a bore, but he was worse than that, he was a genuine threat to me. He represented danger in that he not only intended to take my daddy away from me, but he also had the power to do it. He wasn't even bothering to be covert or cunning; he had faith in his beauty, in their past history and in some vulnerable part of Daddy that I had not seen until now and which appalled me.

On the day of Mandy's arrival Jimmy drove us to a restaurant in the King's Road. It described itself as a bistro. I sat in the front of the car for the first time in my life, smoking Jimmy's cigarettes furiously and making dark plans in which Mandy suffered and I triumphed and one of us – not me – ended up looking like beef jerky. Mandy, meanwhile, sat in the back speaking Spanish to Daddy and worse, far worse, Daddy answered fluently.

I began to regret having done German O level, which I had only taken anyway to annoy my grandmother and thereby remind her that I was alive. It was a simple ruse, regularly implemented but without result. Granny, blind to anyone except herself, was the consummate narcissist. She may also have been a sociopath. It's miraculous that I turned out as well as I did. Her logic, as I think I have established, was unconstricted by normal perceptions. To her mind a person who learned to speak German was a person who was training to run Dachau. I tried to introduce Otto Dix and Günter Grass to the discourse. I showed her pictures and expounded on Expressionism but I was alone in my views. She simply walked around the house with her thin legs in a goose step. Then she fell down the stairs doing it so that was that for a bit. Tubigrip on the ankle, walking stick in one hand, gin and it in the other.

Anyway. German was of no use to me during this particular scene of horror. Mandy and Daddy spoke Spanish to each other and Daddy was beginning to turn into somebody I didn't know. I was hurt and confused.

Mandy ate as if it was his last meal. There was a lot of theatrical dabbing of the mouth with a starched white napkin, which had begun the evening in the shape (appropriately) of a Torquemada mask.

I knew that Mandy was a girl from the streets. You, my friend, I thought to myself, were a starving child, but a beautiful one. You have always fucked men for money. I wonder if you're aware that you will not be able to so for ever. I wonder if my Daddy is your last mark. That you are hoping that he will marry you and provide you with the security that you will never be able to provide for yourself.

'*El vino, es muy rico!*' he said several times during the four courses. He sent one of his three glasses back to be washed and studied himself, without shame, in the knife, making his lips into a moue as he did so.

I laughed out loud.

Mandy glared at me.

Daddy looked at me as if I were a stranger who had to sit with them because the restaurant was crowded. 'What's so funny?'

'Nothing.' I glared at him with incandescent fury but he didn't notice.

My instincts, alerted to danger, had removed the appetite in order to prepare the body to fight. I was not hungry. I thought I would never be hungry again.

Daddy stared at Mandy with undisguised love in his eyes. I couldn't believe it. I had had three years of his undivided attention and now, without warning, I was being abandoned. I was staring at the train as it was leaving the station. Fight or flight? Fight. Somebody was going to be thrown out of this hellhole of a nest and it was not going to be me. Sibling rivalry had settled on my psyche.

I went to the loo, took down my pants, and put them in my handbag. My dress – a pinafore shift in black wool with two white buttons in the front and a dear little pleat at the side – was short, 1960s short. It wasn't mucking about. The hemline was six inches below my waist – it wasn't as small as a tennis skirt but it could have been a tunic. When I bent over this is what you saw: two full round cheeks, smooth and white, the dark crevice of my arse, the top of my thighs, which were tanned and bare, and the hint of the pink lips of a shaved puss. I was wearing knee-high black patent leather boots, very tight on the calves, with rounded toes and three-inch heels. I knew what I was doing. Of course, I did. It was a simple animal presentation – the baboon buttock – the primal sign of receptivity.

I stepped smartly back into the restaurant. Daddy smiled at me vaguely as if he had left his glasses at home.

'Oops.' I allowed the contents of my handbag to shower in a noisy clatter onto the floor – lipsticks, money, knickers, Smarties, address book, keys, apple, Mason and Pearson hairbrush, six pairs of shades, a book about James Hunt. All over the floor.

Well.

They all had to be slowly collected by a bare-arsed broad on all fours with no pants on and her dress halfway up her back.

Daddy, emerging at last from his irritating coma, bent down, picked up the hairbrush and gave it to me with a meaningful look, which sent the wet straight to my naked mons. 'Behave yourself. And go and put your pants back on, at once.'

I ignored him. I was beginning to really enjoy myself. I stayed on all fours, pushed my buttocks up and crawled around on the floor of the restaurant slowly retrieving my possessions. Some of them had rolled quite far, which meant that I had to crawl under other people's tablecloths and retrieve items from a jungle of ankles and brogues and Gucci courts. I found other things on the way, a five-pound note being one of them, and a keyring in the shape of a golf ball.

My eye line was low so I could only guess at the effect that this performance was having. I expected that my bare bottom was being well received and I would emerge to a stand-up ovation from the entire restaurant.

Docking, finally, at the next-door table in order to find that last item, I found myself face to face with a hand holding my pants. 'Here,' said a voice. 'I expect these are yours.'

I stood up, hair over my face, dust all over my legs, slightly flushed in the face, to see a man aged about 25. I tugged my dress over my thighs, rather unnecessarily in the circumstances. 'You can keep them if you like,' I said.

'Much obliged.' He put them in his pocket.

I reinserted myself in the seat at our table and was pleased to note that I was being watched, overtly and covertly, by every man within visibility.

Except one.

He was staring into a hard brown face and asking it if it would like a glass of dessert wine.

I put my hand on Daddy's lap. He was hard. Very hard. I could feel the tough flesh under my fingers, the warm root, ready and erect. But it wasn't for me. He didn't slap me away, but he did remove my hand firmly and place it on the top of my own thigh.

I lost it. A lawyer would have described it as temporary madness.

The sweet trolley arrived, laden with a pyre of profiteroles, various tarts and gateaux and a glass bowl full of floating fruits. Daddy never ate pudding – he liked port and stilton – but I always did. I would rather have had just the pudding actually, and when on my own only ate ice cream and cake. Mandy was the same, a sugar eater and a slut. We had something in common then.

He pointed to the Black Forest gateau, which was often on offer in the bistros of yore. It was multilayered and decorated with swirls of whipped cream and chocolate hundreds and thousands. I seem to remember that jam was involved as well.

The dessert wine was poured into one of a cluster of glasses. Mandy tucked his napkin into his tight white T-shirt, and was aiming his fork from a height in order to turf the glutenous brown pile that was his chocolate cake.

I rose to my feet and pulled the edge of the tablecloth as hard as I could. I didn't know what would happen, but I was sure there would be gratifying noise and chaos.

There was.

Glasses, plates, candlesticks, ashtrays, cutlery, cruets – all flew into the air and smashed onto the floor with a great cacophony of shattering and clattering.

Revenge was a dish served cold and in the lap.

Mandy's plate of chocolate cake tipped up and fell face down onto his tight white jeans so that he looked as if he had had a terrible accident, the nature of which one suspects the police have to deal with when patrolling the streets when the pubs have shut.

Daddy got a glass of port in his crotch.

He leaped to his feet. 'Christ, Stella.'

I left the party.

Who knows if this was the right thing to do or not, and who cares? I felt much much better. I felt happy. I felt excited. I was to spend many hours playing it over in my mind and enjoying every second of it. I still think of it as being one of my finest moments, a career peak if you will.

The man who had been sitting at the next-door table followed me onto the street. 'Are you all right?'

He was thin and earnest. Ernest Hemingway. His hair had been influenced by Spandau Ballet and was a dark quiff arrangement. He was wearing eye make-up and green nail polish and black leather trousers. He was tall and white and not at all bad. He was also my age, which I hadn't experienced for many months, having allowed myself to be confined in the world of Daddy. But I was aware that somewhere out there my peer group were up to something. I saw them peering out of magazines. The men were all dandified and ruffled and immaculately made up; the women, like female starlings, were of duller appearance and weaker song.

'I've been better,' I replied, looking up at him.

'Would you like to go for a drink?'

I wanted Daddy to make me kneel by the side of his bed. I wanted to take his stiff cock wherever he wanted to push it. I wanted him to kiss my neck all night. But he was going to do these things with Mandy. A man named Mandy. A supercilious epicene would be where I should be.

'OK.'

'I'm Stephen.'

The truth is that I would not have remembered his name had I not recounted these details in my diaries. I still have a Polaroid, one of the many he took in his flat that night. He took a series of my boots and legs. He was a graphic designer.

Stephen had a flat in Ladbroke Grove, which, in those days, was the frontline and only inhabited by those who did not mind the idea of being stabbed to death. It would be difficult to stab Stephen to death – he was very tall, he walked very fast, he wore a flapping woollen cape with a big clasp at the neck and he carried a cane with a silver skull. An assailant would have to be either very brave or very stoned to take him on. He shared his accommodation with a man who, when we arrived in the sitting room, was face down on the sofa trying to unzip himself down the back of a vintage Balenciaga ballgown. 'I'm stuck!' he yelled. 'Get me out of this!'

He was a graphic designer as well. Amongst other things. Stephen unzipped him. The man gathered up the cloud of cream taffeta and netting and went to bed saying he was exhausted and everything was a nightmare. I knew what he meant.

Stephen's body was long and white and he had an average-sized dick. This was disappointing after Daddy but I was polite, as I always am, knowing that kindness in these situations is the best way to maintain an erection.

There was a picture of Adam Ant above his bed and 'Bela Lugosi is Dead' on the turntable. It was an era when fairy lights and religious imagery were the motifs of bohemian existence. Stephen and his flatmate were the masters of the found objet and Portobello Road panache so there were kitsch Kens and devils and some strange outsider artefacts made by their friends. A necklace, huge and clunky, had been threaded from egg cups and trolls. A collage had been constructed from hooker call cards. There was a poster for Kenneth Anger's *Scorpio Rising*. And everywhere there were piles of Polaroids and books by Aleister Crowley and flyers about Psychic TV; Nietzsche appeared on the dusty bookshelf. Always. Neitzsche. Unread yes. Understood no.

I pointed out to myself that it was pointless trying to codify the chaos; philosophers had tried and committed suicide when they had discovered that it was pointless.

I was a bit drunk, or squiffy as my grandmother used to say when the police brought her back. I tried not to think of chaos, which, at that moment, was Daddy and Mandy.

Stephen poured some red wine into two silver goblets and lit about thirty church candles so that the dramatic chiaroscuro stained the red walls darkly, throwing light onto a stuffed bargain basement otter and making its eyes look evil, like the birds in the Bates Motel. Bauhaus changed to the hollow angst of Andrew Eldritch – 'pain looks great on

other people that's what they're there for'. Stephen seemed
to agree. He was divesting himself. Languidly removing his
white body from its loose black cerements. I half expected
a crow to fly out from one of the dark folds.

In the bedroom there were Jesuses, or Jesi as I expect they
are known in the plural. Their pink faces glowed with the
baroque misery of the crucifixion as the candles flickered
over the reds and black and into a full-length mirror. He lay
down on his bed. It had a cast-iron head in which he had
twisted mangled toys, dried flowers and black lace. Eldritch
became a Gregorian chant and then Siouxsie Sioux and then
back to Marian – some lugubrious goth pall-bearer must
have mashed a tape up for him. His dick stood up as a white
stick in the middle of the black froth of his pelvis.

I unbuttoned my black minidress. It slid smoothly over
my breasts, down my legs and into a pool on the floor. I
stood in front of him, naked except for my shiny black
boots. My make-up was smudged and my hair was mussed.
There were bruises on the top of my arms where Daddy had
pinched me. I think I had refused to kiss him. I like being
pinched, though it's not my favourite sensation in the
spectrum of pain.

I played with my tits and licked my lips. I was ready to
go anywhere.

Stephen stared at me with pleasure. He was a designer,
after all. 'You look amazing,' he said. 'I have never met a
girl who shaves her bush completely. It's great. I love it. It's
so weird!'

Moving slowly from the bed, he stood in front of me, so
that we were pelvis on pelvis, his gristle on my smooth baby
lips. He sucked my nipples and nibbled them. Then, without
warning, he dropped onto his knees and kissed my boots.

'You can slap me in the face if you like,' he said.

I slapped him in the face.

I slapped him as if he was the abandoning daddy. Hard. You could have heard the crack in the next borough. The right side of his pale cheek flushed up into a red stain. His dark-blue eyes started to glitter. He looked up at me. He was naked and vulnerable. I didn't know how much he could take, how much he wanted to take. I moved into the place where sexual cruelty is requested and the giver must take responsibility for accessing a dangerous part of themselves. In order to meet his needs and give him pleasure, I had to control the ebb and flow of disassociation.

This was to stand on the edge of a primal cruelty whose existence amongst the animal instincts is usually explained through the ancient needs of survival. It was to play with Mirbeau's contention, in *The Torture Garden*, that everything, in the end, is about murder: 'We attenutate physical violence by giving it a legalised outlet: industry, colonial trade, war, the hunt or anti-semitism, because it is dangerous to abandon oneself to it immoderately and outside the law.'

The more a man prostrates himself the nearer I am to killing him. I risk being subsumed by the compulsion to cut and strangle and walk away. Men with masochistic tendencies tend to want the same range of stimuli, which is why, if you ever survey this market, the items on sale are all the same. There is a universality of symbols and triggers and archetypes. Human sexuality, like the blues, has few notes and many tunes. Latex, rubber, fur, heels, mother underwear, nylon, cartoon breasts, whips, Amazonian women, powerless men, teachers, nurses, nannies, chains, cells, bars, medical equipment, humiliation, scat, piss. A pro-dom hooker only has to learn three lines.

The submissive wants slapping and whipping and tying and nipple torture; he does not (usually) want a glass in his face or a blade down his back. Sadism is not my métier; I do not like the stress that it provokes in the dreadful recesses of the psyche, the id if you will – where survival instincts lurk and all the thoughts that have escaped morality. I am not excited by that. But I am elevated by the idea of universal revenge. When a man asks to be kicked about, or flogged, or hurt, in the name of his pleasure zone, I find myself avenging the wrongs of history. It is easy for me to see the naked body in front of me as the symbol of the gender, and just as easy to blame that gender for all the extraordinary evil. I think of the stake. I think of Rwanda. I think of the Stalags. I think of Fred West. I did not understand Them. I did not understand how *They* can be criminals and artists and scientists and saints and dictators and football yobs.

Did Daddy feel these things about me? Did he have to lose respect for me in order to please me? When I abnegated responsibility and stayed young did he lose sight of me? Did he feel like killing me when he beat me? Were our games making barriers and that was why he was finding it so easy to walk away from me?

Perhaps I had hidden myself so well that the woman had disappeared leaving only a shadowy character with no presence. Daddy did not think of me as his important little darling, but some hooker toy, easily expended with. Certainly he seemed to have no idea of the power of the emotional bonds that he had helped us weave between each other. His behaviour was extrarordinary, cruel and unforgivable. I felt like beating Stephen but I wanted to beat Daddy and Mandy, particularly if it caused them no pleasure. Stephen made it clear that a whipping would cause him much pleasure and that he did not receive nearly enough of this type of attention in his life, despite mingling with an underworld of subcultural outsiders wearing white gloves, pan make-up and a small semblance of higher education and thoughts of radicalism.

I did not dislike Stephen, but neither did I care about him. I knew what would thrill him and I could fulfil his idea of foreplay, but it was not from any generosity or affection, it was a cold experiment to assess my own limits – to test where I could go, what I could do, and whether I had the skills to do it. Dreadful really. I feel quite ashamed when I think of it. I won't go to Heaven, but then I never really wanted to, it being a nightclub full of boys in gold shorts.

Stephen, like me, was exerting a self-centered pursuit of pleasure. It was he who knelt down in front of me and handed over the leather belt, the belt a skull head. His dick pumped up, his body was desperate for the feel of the lash. I looked down at him and kicked him over onto the floor where he lay whitely. I decided against a leather belt as I did not have the confidence that I could carry it off, having had no experience with it. These things require some skill, after all, and my hands are small. It might have been a violent fiasco rather than an exquisite interlude.

'Got any rope?' I asked.

'No. There are scarves over there.'

'Get them.'

He brought me a tin with Elvis on it and offered it to me. I extricated a vintage Dior scarf and tied his hands behind his back. 'Lie face down on the bed and do not speak unless I tell you that you may.'

He did as he was told.

I placed a pillow under his stomach so that his arse was raised and presented to me as an easy target. I looked at it with some pleasure. I love bottoms. I just do. Male or female. I love their round shape and smooth skin. I could stare at them all day.

Stephen was silent, perhaps going somewhere old and young where punishment had once been meted out to him. I knew this tension, of course, having waited for Daddy so many times. I knew that the imagination started to take over and the body started to prepare and that it was exciting and frightening.

I surveyed his room for an appropriate tool for punishment and found a wooden ruler on his desk. Perfect.

'This is going to hurt,' I commented.

He groaned in the pleasure of anticipation and writhed.

I brought the ruler down hard on his bare cheeks.

It made a red line and he yelped.

I reached under his pelvis and felt his dick; it was hard and it was twitching.

We were on the right track.

I brought the ruler down again right on the white target making another crimson streak.

Then again six more times, slightly harder each time.

He screamed and shouted and writhed.

I wondered if he would cry. I hoped not. I had never seen a man cry and did not wish to start now.

I decided he had not had enough and brought the ruler down again six more times. I knew it would be really hurting by now, as Daddy had done this often enough to me. Not as hard, I don't think, though I wasn't sure of my own strength in this scenario. I could only judge the effect from the lividity of the flesh and the reaction of the groaning man.

I stopped for a minute, and felt the burning flesh. I inserted my hands beneath his buttocks to the soft root of his balls and the perineum. I softly massaged them, stroking his pleasure centres, telling him that I was pleased that he was hard and that I expected him to stay that way because he was going to have to please me. Then I pushed my finger reassuringly into his rectum .

'No, please,' he begged. 'I'll come.'

'You had better not.'

Then I spanked him because I felt like it. I smacked him hard on top of his flaming cheeks and he went into a second wave of pain, lost now in endorphins and confusion and pleasure.

'Get up,' I instructed. 'Get up.'

I untied his wrists and made him lie on his back.

I sat astride him.

'Stella . . .'

'Be quiet.' I put my hand over his mouth.

Slowly, I eased myself up and down on him, my wet labia kissing the surface of his shaft, caressing every throbbing purple vein on it, until I saw that he was leaking.

'Don't you dare come,' I said, slapping him in the face.

'I want to. I want to.'

I got off him.

He yelled out loud. Then said, 'No, please, please carry on! I want to be in you.'

'You will wait for me,' I said. 'And if you don't I will beat you again.'

I slapped him in the face and spat at him.

I slid myself down on him again, and took him slowly into me. I took my time and it served him right. I took him deep inside me, feeling all of him all the way up, until some inner response was triggered and a subtle internal spasm shuddered through me, surprisingly emotional. It took me by surprise, as a rush of gratitude and love flooded through me, gratitude and love for a good hard dick but not for a man I did not know. They were two different things, things that one could not know when in the throes, the dangerous moment when one is subsumed. There are a few fleeting dangerous seconds when one thinks, He is the one, I want this inside me for the rest of my life. He cannot leave me. If He goes I will be nothing. I will enter the void and I will die.

I jerked myself off him and as I did so he exploded onto his stomach. I watched politely, knowing how proud they are of their seed. God knows they have spread enough of it about, judging by the world population figures.

I untied him. He tried to hug me. I allowed a kiss on the lips.

'That was amazing,' he said. 'Thank you.'

'You're welcome,' I said primly.

'Please may I kiss your tits.'

'No,' I said, and put my dress back on.

I left him twisted around as he attempted to survey the red stripes on his buttocks in a full-length mirror. His dick was semi-tumescent. I could have had him again if I had wanted to but I didn't want to. I wanted Daddy.

After that, Stephen was my slave. He was always ringing me up and offering himself. We drove around. He had an old burgundy Rover with Roman Catholic crucifixes hanging from the mirror. We fucked a bit, laughed enough. He picked me up when and where I told him to and left when I told him to. He once came all the way to Bermondsey to collect me. Do not ask me what I was doing there, I do not know. Do not ask me where Bermondsey is, I do not know. Stephen, like most men, could read a map. He was also self-employed which is closely related to unemployed. He had time on his hands, which he enjoyed devoting to my requirements. He was always hard and there is something to be said for that.

He thought he loved me and he was very good at massages, but the awful truth was that, though well read and basically kind, he was a bit of a bore. He didn't have many ideas of his own. Still, he was an excellent chauffeur, a good masseur, a satisfactory fuck, and I didn't mind whipping his arse for him.

The tall goth unleashed the diva in me. I became quite the dominatrix, although it always felt as if I had taken the wrong coat home. I enjoyed his long white shaft with its glowing pink bobble! Sometimes I knotted it up in rope, which he liked and was a first for me. I didn't mind giving him a good slapping, it was a distraction. In the end, though, I didn't want a slave. Being a mistress bored me. I was bereft.

I wanted Daddy. I never told Stephen that because I am not bad-mannered. Anyway he was involved in his own needs, he saw me as his mistress, the marvellous and all-powerful matriarch of his own fantasy. He did not see me – a little girl who had lost her daddy for the second time in her life. He saw me as the figure he had invented in his own present. He did not see my past. He did not care about any of my other aspects. He did not care what made me. That's the problem with games, I guess. Nobody knows who anybody really is. This is not necessarily a bad thing, but it is a thing.

I, having grown up with a volatile madwoman, knew how to be aware of danger. I was conscientious in my investigations and attuned to peripheral vision. I tended to learn about people in case I had to protect myself against them. I knew that Stephen's father was a doctor in Leeds, his mother was a teacher and he had a sister called Stacey. I knew that he had read most of the classics.

I could not work out whether his self-esteem was very high or very low. He seemed fairly stable, but he did smoke quite a lot of pot. He adored me, which was very gratifying, and it eased the pain of daddy desertion.

I did not know why he was a masochist and neither did he. He said he was prone to dark thoughts and needed to get away from them. A hiding served that purpose and released some of the guilt that he felt from leaving his old parents to look after themselves in their depressing semi-detached while he cavorted about London and enjoyed himself.

'I find it difficult to enjoy myself,' he said, 'despite the fact that I am not religious.'

Stephen suggested I get a tattoo on my cunt and I agreed. He said he wanted to kiss the blood on it when it had first been made. He said he would cream my puss with healing creams and look after my shaved baby mons until the design healed. Then he wanted to take photographs, lots of them, in colour and in close-up, which he planned to blow up to the size of posters and make into some weird art series.

Tattoos were not mainstream fashion in 1985 – they were still the symbology of the outsider. Tattoos were worn by some punk rockers, many undiagnosed self-harmers, category-C inmates, geriatric sailors, suburban pikeys, Santa Monica boulevardiers and Coleherne queens. The straights had not started to modify themselves, so the tat still had some significance as a statement of self-identification.

Stephen, being a true masochist, had a back full of homages to the god Pan. He looked like the cover of a Blue Oyster Cult album.

I went to a bizarre salon in Soho and chose a design – a tiny scorpion.

'Take about two hours,' said the hirsute artisan behind the till. 'Where do you want it?'

'On my cunt,' I answered, staring him down.

A moist tongue flicked pinkly over through the foliage of his beard and his beringed fingers played on top of the counter as if he was practising the piano. Two calm blue eyes stared unblinking from the hairy face. I thought of Animal in the Muppets.

'Mmm. I did that for a stripper last year. Shouldn't be a problem. You might have to get a taxi home – could be uncomfortable for a couple of days.'

I rang Stephen. 'I need you here now.'

'Yes Mistress.'

Stephen arrived like Batman, accompanied by screeching tyres and a flapping cape. He leaped dramatically into the salon.

'Everything all right?'

'Yes. Wait there and don't jig about.'

'Can't I watch?'

'It's all right with me,' said the beard, shrugging.

I removed my miniskirt and pastel-pink cotton panties but left my ankle socks and stilettos on for Stephen's pleasure as I am, in the end, a kind person, considerate even.

Straddling like a slut below the tattooist, I spread out on the couch and pointed to my bald puss.

'There,' I said, indicating the spot a little above the line where my pubic hair would grow back and which, with a certain style of underwear, or bikini bottom, could be revealed when I wished it to be.

Availing myself of this display was a very unpleasant and painful experience rendered worse by the fact that, like most masochists, I have a very low resistance to actual physical pain. And I had to pretend to two staring men that I was all right.

I was left with a red mark at the top of my pubic bone and no indication of the venomous creature underneath. I felt as if my fanny had been burned with a blow torch. I handed over the limp bank notes with some resentment.

Stephen helped me into the car and made appreciative noises all the way back to Chelsea. At this point the endorphins kicked in good and proper, my fanny lit up with pain and need, my head dazed with self-satisfaction. Once in the flat I got on all fours on the bed and made Stephen roger me slowly from the back.

I liked my scorpion. When it emerged from the scab it was small and neat and beautifully detailed. It represented freedom from Daddy, and a revenge on him, as it was an immoveable symbol of my ability to enact enterprise without his permission. I relished the thought of telling him what I had been up to and seeing his reaction. He would be furious.

He thought body modification was immature, an unnecessary outlet for freaks and losers and pop stars who had received no formal education and didn't understand Latin.

Stephen knew the rudiments of black magic – in that he had some books by Genesis P-Orridge and a silver pentacle that had been charged by a warlock in Glastonbury. He influenced me with ideas about these powers. Stephen said sex magic worked though, when pressed, he couldn't provide any convincing evidence for this being true. I couldn't resist trying. I'll try anything, me, except snails. He would put his finger in me, wipe the juice over a black candle and place it in the middle of a pentacle. He would mutter incantations of Kabbalic principle and I would sit there with a joint, my heart thudding, my reality askew, praying hard for my daddy to come back to me.

Once, when I had smoked one too many, I had a paranoid vision where Daddy came back to me when I was an old woman, Baby Jane, only a punk version with black hair and purple lips and the desiccation of age etched into features twisted by disappointment.

Resolutely and with passion, I muttered incantations to the dark side, begging for solution, wanking for Daddy, climaxing to thoughts of his return, begging him to come back to me.

Finally he rang.

'Where have you been? I've been trying to get hold of you for weeks.'

'Mind your own business.'

'I miss my naughty girl.'

'I don't like you any more.'

'Nonsense. I want to see you. Meet me in Fortnum's tomorrow at four thirty.'

'What about that other . . . thing?'

'It'll just be us. I'll see you at four thirty.'

In the past he would have said don't be late or there'll be trouble, but he didn't. I took this as a sign that he no longer loved me.

This brings me to the L word.

Love.

How little I knew about it. How little I knew of its incredible complexity and unfathomable aspects. I had no idea that forgiveness was involved, or hate was in there, alongside boredom, compromise, irritation, disappointment, disillusion, frustration, did I say boredom?

I only knew love as sex and need. I knew love as the endless hope of filling unfillable gaps. Looking back, now, twenty years later, I am the same age as Daddy was when I met him. I am nearly fifty. I am surprised I did not drive him mad with my self-centred needs, which I thought were important and meaningful. I guess the theory is that you only have your reality and he had enough patience and wisdom to see my defects and love me anyway.

How little one knows. I thought I knew everything. I thought I was a sophisticate attuned to the requirements of modernity. I played with my body and psyche as if they were recreational drugs.

Drama and intensity, positive and negative, highs and lows, these were passion and passion was love. I was not bored and I like to think that I was not boring.

Daddy was not afraid of the L word and he often told me that he loved me, even when we weren't in bed. If you are gagging a girl and whipping her arse, it's important to love her, I think, or say you do at least. I couldn't bend over for someone, take the pain and buggery and then walk away without the affection and aftercare that, at that moment in my life, I thought was love.

Now he had betrayed me and hate had arrived; grief and love and shock and hate, all at once, thanks to the man called Mandy.

Kevin the hairdresser said that Mandy was short for Mandrax but I think he was only being supportive. I wanted to hurt Daddy back but I did not know how to. I did not know the nature of my power over him, or, indeed, whether I had any. I did not know the truth of his vulnerability; he had only revealed daddy care, never the chinks in the armour of the actual man.

He always seemed invulnerable, physically healthy as he was, erect in stature and large of dick; he was rich, clever and confident. But then I wanted him to be these things and they may have been figments of my imagination. I could have been the sum of mad delusions – he might have been a sick fuck with clinical issues and a penchant for disco queens.

I didn't care. I wanted him back. He was mine. I needed him. I was his little girl and I could not live without him. Every day that he was absent was a long day where the hours were only there to be breathed before the cocktail hour, memory lapse and collapse.

I spent 24 hours preparing myself to reunite with Daddy. I assumed that he wanted a meeting because he wanted to continue to see me on some level. He wanted me to step back into his life and my position had to be renegotiated. I hoped that Mandy had packed his bags and gone but I doubted it. Street hustlers onto a good thing don't leave until the police arrive.

How much of Mandy could I take? How accommodating could I be in order to win what I needed, wanted and loved?

I made myself ready for Daddy.

Black fringe, big eyes, red lipstick that he liked to smudge off with his hands leaving a red mark on my cheeks and chin. Tight white capri pants with no knickers so that the orbs of the female bottom could be seen clear and round and begging for administration. Leopard-skin stilettos in which I could hardly walk, teamed with a vintage leopard-skin handbag, round with a handle at the top. A tiny tight eau de Nil cotton T-shirt that accentuated the narrowness of my shoulders and the perkiness of my tits. Finally, I shrouded myself with Stephen's leather jacket under which one could hide and from which one could growl. Daddy would hate the leather jacket and I wanted him to hate it. He would think it was too big and masculine and where had I got it from anyway? That jacket was as good as actually wearing a badge saying, 'I am sleeping with someone else, put that in your pipe and smoke it.'

The hair? The hair was in two darling dark little pigtails.

7. 1986

Fortnum's. Fortnum's, lovely Fortnum's.
   Old fashioned and stylish and serene. I could sing a
song about you but I will rein myself in for the sake of
narrative.

Oh God, there he was behind the menu. Crisp white shirt,
dark trousers, black brogues, cheekbones, dark hair occasionally flopping over the forehead in the way that belied his
age and occasionally had to be pushed back when he was
tense. I loved him. He still made my heart beat. He still
made me wet. As I wove through the tables of the Fountain
café I could feel it happening between my legs. By the time
I sat down I had melted completely.

He had ordered already so I didn't have any stressful
decisions to make. He knew I liked cucumber sandwiches
and a chocolate milkshake and I knew that I would be
expected to eat the sandwiches first. He looked at me
meaningfully when they arrived, decorated with a single
sprig of cress. Luckily they were crustless and small and
triangular because my stomach was a nut.

Overcome, I nibbled the bread and looked down into my lap. I had no experience of this kind of thing – of truth and mature conversations and being put on the spot with what my grandmother called 'all that'. I was not advantaged by insight. Ignorant and inarticulate as I was, my only form of expression was through my sexuality. I spoke through my body. I did not know how to process feelings; I did not have the language or the technique; I hardly knew what feelings were. When they arose in all their heat and confusion, they subsumed me with mortification. I was paralysed by them unless I was naked and in bed. And, at that point, of course, I was not. I was in a tea room that had been established in 1800 and something and employed the most charming staff in London.

So there we were, young and old. I hardly knew him. I had lost my confidence. I didn't know what to say.

He spoke. Men. They like to, don't they? They like speaking. Never draw breath some of them.

I was glad he did. I couldn't and, even if I could, I suspect I would have kept silent. Silence, in my small experience, was an effective defence and an effective act of provocation. Daddy had slapped me for it in the past. He recognised it for what it was, a need for attention, a need to move the scene forward and a part of foreplay. 'Look at me.'

I folded my arms and looked at him.

The years were falling away. I was twenty, then twelve, then eight, then seven. I kicked the table leg.

'Don't do that.'

I felt like kicking his leg but I didn't.

He put his hand across the white tablecloth and took mine. One defence down. 'I'm sorry I didn't tell you,' he said. 'I wasn't lying. The subject just didn't seem to come up. Then Mandy arrived out of the blue. I haven't seen him since 1977. I don't know how he found me actually.

Anyway I can't turn him away, he's on his uppers. He can't go home and he's penniless. He has no one.'

Penniless? I thought. He was wearing his body weight in gold jewellery. And why can't he go home?

'In general I prefer to sleep with women, and I certainly prefer to talk to them, but I have always been drawn to male beauty and have enjoyed it since boarding school.'

Ah. Boarding school. It was bound to come up. Daddy told me that the years during which he received a private education were the worst of his life and it had taken him a long time to recover. I knew he wasn't the only one. My cousin Danny went to Eton, washed his hands for three weeks and had to be taken away in an ambulance.

Daddy's father had repaired to South Africa in order to invest in a diamond mine but mainly in order to avoid his wife, who he disliked intensely, an opinion in which he was not alone. Daddy's mother bred pugs. She was not present either physically or emotionally. So Daddy was left at prep school and public school and beaten at both. Isolated and friendless, he was made to clean the boots of some revolting older boy who alternately caned him and kissed him.

The older boy was an awe-inspiring beauty, according to Daddy. Everyone was in love with him and to attract his attention at all was to lift oneself out of the shameful mire of ignominy suffered by any twelve year old experiencing an education system designed by the criminally insane.

'I have never been buggered,' he suddenly said quite loudly and to the surprise of the distinguished Polish émigré who was in the middle of serving him a cup of tea. 'I liked kissing men and fondling them, I liked feeling their bodies and looking at their faces, but I could never actually take them inside me. Either it hurt me or they didn't want to or anyway, it never happened.

'I liked them licking me though, my balls, my arse, I liked them licking me everywhere.'

The gentleman waiter slipped away as if he was a joke pound note being jerked by an invisible thread.

'What about the other way around?'

'Oh. That happened. Very enjoyable.'

So Daddy became quite promiscuous in that he slept with everybody who asked him to and then, later, at Cambridge, indulged in the femme frills of the 1960s and slept with men and women there too. He was dark, he was gaunt, he was looming, he was damaged. Women adored him; men wanted him.

'I have been involved with more women than men,' he said.

'But men have been in my life. I can't really see that there is anything I can do about it.' He was right, of course. There is nothing you can do about your sexual tastes. They are hard wired. History has proved that if nothing else.

'If I find them beautiful, I find them beautiful. You know what I mean, surely. You have slept with women?'

'I suppose so.' I have slept with women, not because I was transported by their beauty, but, usually, because they asked me to rather than any particular effort made by myself. I slept with women because I liked doing things I had not done before and finding out things I did not know. There was always the slim chance that an intense physical experience would draw up some recall from the past that could serve to illuminate the present and clarify the consistent confusion that often overwhelmed me. So, yes, I did sleep with women. I slept with women who looked like men, who rode motorbikes and owned spanners, and who knew what to do with a dildo. I liked big ugly male women which, according to the lesbian directive of the time, meant I was not a lesbian.

I did not want to draw in other players, male or female, gay or repressed. I wanted him to myself because, at this point, he was the only person with whom I was involved and in whom I was interested. He, however, did not share this. I was not enough. He had done me and he was bored. He had become bored before I did and that was a first for me. I am always bored first.

I felt like standing on the table and asking him where I stood but I didn't. Even in that callow era of my shallow life I knew I was not destined for convention. I knew that I could not talk in the way that women's magazines suggest because I did not want any of the prizes that are the accepted interpretation of modern life. I was never going to be a wife or mother; I did not want durable consumer goods; I knew that night creams could not retain the youth of the skin. I was blessed with a precocious distrust of lies. I was not afraid of the future and I certainly wasn't afraid of death. These things, I was to learn, were unusual. They gave me the strengths that I had, but they did not provide the capability to articulate them.

I could not negotiate with Daddy because I had no identifiable plan. I did not see myself ending up anywhere. I could not see myself committing, so I had no demand except to be loved for myself and enjoy things. I could not then negotiate demands. I could not talk about 'us' because I was cursed with the knowledge that in the great scheme of things there could be no convincing definition because all relationships were subject to impermanence.

For most women this impermanence is staunched by the need to breed and that basic instinct introduces necessary confinement. But if you did not need to breed you were not dancing to the theme that played in the majority's lives. These modernist thoughts, enlightened though they were, did not repress the dark and uncontrollable venoms that are the sure result of not getting exactly what one wants. I still wanted Daddy.

I was Daddy's girl.

I wanted him to myself.

I wished that Mandy was dead.

I lurched into the greater need of the child. The sandwiches were dry, the milkshake cold and clammy; it was too much. I knew that I could not, at this point, walk out of his life and stay out of it. It would hurt and not in nice way. I had to stay with him, on his terms, dreadful though they were.

I wondered if I had any power to hurt him. I wondered if he would be as terrified by my departure as I was by the idea of his. I suspected not. He had once told me that emotions change with age; you don't care so much about anything, you are frightened by less, you have less joy and less anxiety.

I knew what I wanted at this slow moment amongst the white tablecloths and silver teapots and women down from Hampshire for dinner and a show. I wanted him to do as I said. I wanted him to say things like, 'If you leave me I will fly all over the world and bring you back. I want you and only you with me for the rest of my life. I will prevent illness and poverty and loneliness.'

I played my cards close. 'Well, you won't mind what I do,' I said, 'now what we laughingly call our relationship seems to be open to the public.'

Daddy swallowed, looked sad and shrugged. It was the first time I had seen him shrug; he always had an answer for everything. He shrugged and lost thirty years and I saw the boy who had slept with boys because he was lonely and frightened. I was not ready to see his past or his present. I did not want a human being, I wanted an all-powerful guardian. If he was vulnerable that meant I was too. The perfect mask was showing the face behind it and it made me want to scream out loud.

'You're a paradox, Stella,' he said. 'You want to be safe but you also want danger.'

Ah yes. I am stressed by the insoluble effects of indoctrination – where romantic delusion has infiltrated the psyche from the very first story by Grimm, to every plot and picture and song and graphic image. I was made schizoid by the stress of semiotics and I was not alone. I was not alone in being two women: the one who wanted to be saved by myth and the one driven mad by the knowledge of their own credulity.

Neither of us wanted to leave each other so we went back to my flat in the King's Road. It is quite a messy place, as he pointed out immediately. He said he had seen tidier slums in Naples.

I told him to shut up. He blinked and flushed slightly. But he was still taller than me, and stronger.

I don't really do tidying or cooking and I don't buy things apart from clothes and books. This was evident in the nature of the piles around the place. Piles of clothes, piles of books. A sofa somewhere underneath it all. A nice big bed with a white cover. A kitchen in which there were a couple of apples, some tea, wine and shoes. My diaries were on the kitchen table, in the form of endless scraps of papers and notes and exercise books and pictures, along with felt pens, Biros and Sellotape. I had kept them since I could write. They were and are my hobby. They were and are silly and cryptic and detailed and descriptive and honest. They will always need translation, particularly the ones completed while I was at university and forced to read the unexpurgated Pepys. I made the mistake of creating a code, which took me hours to decipher when I returned to the pages to write this book. There were moons and triangles and numbers which, once translated, revealed irrelevant items about cocktail parties in the New College quad. There were also various items of pervery gleaned from odd moments of shopping and sensual reverie when my mind was on future scenes and what I might do. I went through a stage of frilly knickers and balaclavas, not worn at the same time, for separate occasions. There were a lot of shoes. There was a poster of Pete Murphy and Butler and Wilson tiaras of varying sizes and glitteriness. I wasn't beyond a tutu in those days, though I would never do pastel tights.

'Take your clothes off and lie face down on the bed.'

'Aren't you the little bossy one,' he said. 'You seem to have picked up some tricks.'

'Do it.'

He did as he was told, with some grace. He lay his beautiful white body, long and smooth, along the bed. He was falling into submission and I sensed old pain and old shame and I knew that he wanted them to be released. I suspected he was back at school with old guilt, that unreal and unnecessary emotion, ego-centred and so easily manipulated.

I wanted to hurt him. For the first time I wanted to hurt him. I was not confident that I could inflict any emotional wound, I was not confident of the truth of his affection, but I was confident that, with some ironic permission from him, I could hurt him physically.

'I am going to beat you,' I said.

'I know.'

'You deserve it.'

'I know.'

He was a tall man on a white bed and he was surrendering. I inserted my hands underneath his pelvis and felt his dick. It was semi-tumescent. He was becoming aroused. Fear was not preventing his enjoyment.

I took myself down to black panties, which were a 1950s girdle in their styling, and my push-up black bra. Then I smoothed on a pair of black leather gloves, long, with (real) pearl buttons that he had had made for me, lubed my fingers with KY jelly and pushed them under his nose. 'This is going in you.'

I massaged his balls and his perineum and then slowly inserted my slimy leather finger into his rectum. He loved that. He breathed out with the incipient enjoyment. I massaged some more until he was fully erect. Corporal pain on massive hard-on. What a joy that was going to be for him, but it was going to be accompanied by a punishment that might be hard for him to bear.

I considered dressing him up in some humiliating way, but decided against it. I preferred him naked, naked and vulnerable.

Don't ask me what I was doing with a cane. Things like that came into my life at that time. I seemed to bring it out in people; pervs sense pervs, and people gave me peculiar emblems that they thought would liven things up. I owned various implements of torture and the cane was made of willow, thin and whippy, probably made for a horse rather than a school. 'This will hurt you a lot more than me,' I said.

I brought the cane down on his white buttocks. There was a satisfying swish and it cut a red line across the white flesh.

He yelped and twitched. 'Ow! Jesus. Careful.'

'Shut up.'

I striped him again, and again, red lines striping across the bottom and the thighs. He groaned again and started to breathe heavily.

I stood over him and used all my strength. I went on and on, losing myself in the savagery, watching the tapestry of marks appear, enjoying the groans as they turned into screams.

Then, suddenly, the deep-throated groans of pain turned into manly sobs. His body heaved, he sobbed and he shuddered with the terrifying emotion of release. I had never seen a man cry before and it horrified me. I don't think I had even seen it on the television at that point. I wasn't aware that they could. They can't usually, I suppose, but sometimes they do and he wouldn't stop. Manly crying. Unnerved and returning to a normal space of affection, I dropped the cane, untied him and hugged him, a mother for the first and last time in my life.

His hard-on was huge. I dipped down and licked his helmet gently, telling him that he was a good boy, sucking him with my mouth, teasing him with my tongue, around the edge and the top as I knew he liked it.

Then I sat astride him and fucked him for my own pleasure. All the warm wet internal muscles contracted into a tight sheath, my lower body kissing every nerve on his shaft, caressing every tiny swollen vein. Tighter and tighter I pulled, knowing he could feel every contraction as a kiss on his dick. I pulled the come out of him with my cunt and came as some tip of him connected with some deep internal part of me of which I had no knowledge but was, sometimes unfortunately, wired to gratitude, respect and love. There is nothing like a big dick, my friends.

He ejaculated and I felt the waves of him as he disappeared into the place that men go, losing himself, and groaning deeply as he did so. He lay weak, the tears still on his cheek. I wiped the sweat from his forehead with a clean white flannel.

'What is that on your fanny?' he said.

'A scorpion,' I replied.

I sent him back to Mandy, limp and striped with my own mark. My brand. The livid purple weals that said SB. I had punished Daddy and he was still mine. Mandy wouldn't be getting it that night, at least. There would be a physical distance between them if nothing else.

After that everything entered a new dimension.

I decided to fight.

It could have been fun. Mandy and I could have been friends. We could have enjoyed ourselves under the terms of a mutual agreement, joined by love for Daddy rather than hatred of each other, but we did not.

Mandy had moved into one of the guest rooms at Cheyne Walk so Daddy's lovely white towels were now always damp and stained with fake tan.

They were always out shopping because Mandy needed a shirt, or a facial, or a car or something.

Mandy was manipulative but stupid, which is an unsatis-factory combination. Irritatingly, he did not see me as a threat because he was sure of his own status in the Cheyne domain. He delivered orders to the staff as if he was the newly arrived bride. This drove Jimmy mad. The chauffeur and I would smoke cigarettes in the shrubs, complaining out of the sides of our mouths.

Jimmy, off duty, did not wear his hat and, seeing his face, I realised that he was younger than I had thought, late thirties perhaps. He had the lines and tattoos that reflected a relationship with the criminal justice system, and he had the kind of jaw you sometimes see on men guarding doors at nightclubs or in the background of old Cagney movies. He had a shaved head but his eyes were blue and amused and when not in his uniform he wore alarming crew-necked jerseys that his wife bought for him in Marks & Spencer.

'I don't use the C word often,' he would say, 'but that woman or whatever he is!'

'Do you think he's dangerous?' I asked. 'Kevin the hairdresser told me that he saw him in a club with a knife.'

Jimmy exhaled his smoke thoughtfully. 'Difficult to tell with foreigners, isn't it? Who knows what makes 'em tick? But I seen similar when I was in Coldingley, on drugs charges mainly. Psychos the lot of them.'

Mandy said he was twenty-eight but I suspect he was at least five years older. He had left his sponge bag open once and I noticed that he had two passports, which is all very well, but one bore his photograph with another name. He was always whispering into the phone and he was a fan of club drugs – it was E in the 80s, E and speed as I recall. This should have made Daddy angry but it didn't. He always said he hated drugs but he didn't mind Mandy taking them. I didn't mind Mandy taking them either because it meant he would go to Heaven and leave Daddy and me to play. But this lifestyle left him with comedowns, which he then drank through, and drink was not his friend. Drink brought out the screaming queen. There was smashing and screeching and tears. It was like living with Bette Davis in *Hush . . . Hush, Sweet Charlotte*.

Daddy tried to placate him. He soothed, canoodled and bribed like a mother with a child in a supermarket. If you calm down, you can have this. He had never placated me; but then my tantrums were never real, merely the enactment of foreplay, a way to get his hands on my arse and his mouth on my mouth.

Mandy did not love Daddy. I knew that and it made me livid.

I did watch them having sex, though, and wanked myself off. It was stimulating, two male bodies grinding into each other, all sweat and muscle and violence and admirable erections.

I liked watching Mandy go down on Daddy, I liked watching him submit. Daddy always looked so beautiful naked, I could have watched him doing anything with anyone. His skin was flawless; his body toned without being joke gym queen; his back long and lean, his waist tight, his thighs hard.

Mandy liked me to watch him with Daddy because he thought he was magnificent in bed and my self-esteem would be destroyed by the evidence of this. He thought that by having sex with Daddy without my involvement he was taking Daddy away from me, which was not the case.

Daddy liked me to watch because he liked me to be involved in the situation; he liked me to be there.

I resented sharing. I didn't want to share. I began to see other men. And women. I drew towards leatherwomen in north London, liking their candour and their clothes. I loved my Daddy only, but something shifted. The sex between us became more vanilla as I began to trust him less. I did not want him to dominate me any more. I certainly did not want him to cause me physical pain when the emotional pain was almost too much to bear.

He suggested we all sleep together but I didn't want to. I only wanted to watch. He shaved his balls and cock, which made them look interesting, but I neither fancied nor liked Mandy. Who wanted to kiss that pert little mouth? He smelled terrible. I don't know where he found the cologne from but it pervaded the house like a sickly swamp gas.

I didn't want to enter some blow-job competition where skills were judged as if they were in an eccentric rural show.

I was jealous. I tried to fight it but I could not.

Meanwhile, the more Daddy gave Mandy, the more dangerous he became. He went out all night and slept all day. Lurid figures started to hang out at the house as if they owned it. Drugs arrived and with them a group of young thin girls who liked coke and would do a lot, both to get it and once they had had it. Everything became like an early Martin Amis novel.

Daddy served them cocktails from the silver drinks tray. He was a cross between a father and a butler, playing host to the young things. He gave them lifts, or directed Jimmy to do so. They stayed overnight on his treasured sofas and ate everything out of his fridge. The mornings were ashtrays and the smell of red wine and broken glasses and crumbs on the floor. There was a boy called Rory who wore a Barbour and slept on the stairs. He had Gucci shoes and a habit. I heard him have a fight with Mandy about a silver tray that had disappeared. Silver seemed to be a motif. There was always burned kitchen foil in the downstairs loo.

It should have driven Daddy insane but he didn't seem to mind, didn't seem to notice that they were high and callous and venal.

Some of them were beautiful in an exhumed kind of way, some were beautiful in a blond kind of way. They were all upmarket and lost and driven by the forces of the night because they could not handle the day, the light, the morning, the life. They were spending their parents' money on dancing and drugs. They had no talent, no imagination and no hope.

The youths, feminine and hysterical, saw a rich man in an open house. They thought they had it made and everything was there for the taking. Some of them had the nerve to ask Daddy to lend them money, which he did, if you please, a hundred here a hundred there, he couldn't say no.

Mandy demanded more and more – meals, jewellery, beauty treatments, cash. He was the trophy wife and Daddy was besotted. Driven by the beauty of youth, he was blind to the spoiled mouth, the girly tremolo and the humourless stupidity. Daddy and I no longer went to his house in the country because Mandy did not like to leave London and did not like the country. It scared him and it bored him. There were no shops, he didn't ride, it was cold and damp and he didn't know what to do.

Daddy became more and more dependent on Mandy. He started to do things he would never usually have done. He went to the clubs because he didn't want to let Mandy out of his sight. He would have worn jeans if I hadn't told him he looked absurd. He gave Mandy a credit card because he wanted him to stay. What was his return? An absurd whore who flounced around in itsy-bitsy bikinis, demanding more and more, treating everyone as if they were room service, complaining about everything from the milk in the coffee to the noise in the road, to the weather, to the quality of his hideous yellow cashmere pullover. He would stagger around drunk, knocking Daddy's prized china treasures from their innumerable occasional tables, leaving cigarette burns in the damask, contaminating and polluting.

Mandy spun many yarns about his background. He said he had grown up in an oil barrel in Caracas during the 'revolution'. He had not been to school and it was true that he could not read or write, a fact about which he was strangely proud and mentioned every time we went to a restaurant. He would fling the menu down with a pout and cross his arms over his chest while waiting for Daddy to read out the entire list of starters and entrées while I grew old and withered.

Mandy said he had nearly starved to death as a child. The only food had been supplied by his thirteen-year-old sister who was a prostitute. Mandy, the second of seven, had seen this as a wise career move.

Occasionally, and to my intense amusement, he would claim that he could see into the future due to some ancient gypsy blood on his grandmother's side, a woman, apparently, who could do voodoo and make powerful stews into which various inappropriate species were dropped. 'I see things,' he would announce dramatically. 'I know things. I am senseetive.'

'You must be freezing in those shorts then,' I would say. 'It's November.'

'I will get Jimmeee to turn the 'eating op.'

Little white shorts, buttocks, package, sneakers, short T-shirt, stomach showing, occasionally a roller in the hair, you can imagine it.

Kevin the hairdresser said that to his certain knowledge Mandy had spent two years living with a sixty-year-old businessman on a yacht in the Bahamas. The only reason he was not still there was because there had been a fire. Arson was suspected, the businessman had been unable to claim on the insurance and relations had cooled. Mandy would whine and complain until Daddy took him to Tiffany or Asprey or Hermès and found him the luxury product that would make Mandy happy, though happy is never a word that could be accurately applied to this nasty little man.

Soon he had silver boxes and leather goods and a Rolex watch, which disappeared as quickly as they appeared because Mandy had sold them to buy drugs.

He would occasionally present the newest ring to me with the triumph of a seventeenth-century courtesan.

'That'll set the alarm off in the airport,' I would point out. 'You'll be deported back to Puerto Rico.'

'You stupid bitch,' he would snarl. 'I'm from Venezuela and you know it. Why do you think I have these and you do not? He's bored of you, he wishes you would take that tight little ass out of his sight. He don't like your tutus and your cheapy shades. You think you're Audrey Hepburn, missy, but you're more like Cyndi Lauper. He say you kiss like an ant eater.'

'At least I don't smell like one.'

I didn't think I was Audrey Hepburn, actually. I consider-ed that to be a worse insult than the anteater. I've never been able to stand her voice, her wide eyes or the dancing about the place in flat shoes. Always in black and flitting about, she was worse than a bluebottle. I wished that somebody would bat her away with a rolled-up newspaper.

I liked to think I wasn't like anyone. Daddy always said I was unique and I believed him. He said if I had been an animal I would have been eaten immediately due to the fact that I had no camouflage and would never have a herd to protect me. If I did have the sense to hide in a bush, I would probably spring out just to be annoying.

'You'd be dead in a second,' he observed. 'Your legs would be eaten before sundown.'

'Better dead then dull,' I would note.

'Speaks the naughty girl with a scorpion on her cunt,' he said.

Daddy did not approve of my tattoo. As I had predicted, he took it as a personal slight against him, a symbol of my detachment from his authority. I had had an intense experience that had not involved him. If we had been as we were before Mandy, he would have used it to initiate some exciting scenes, but he knew that in the circumstances of ménage he could not issue these orders with any meaningful authority. Daddy treated Mandy and me as errant children and the more he did so, the more we became locked in a sibling rivalry so intense that it was only a matter of time before somebody was pushed out of the nest and crushed their skull on the ground below. Once, sick and tired of us, he made us both bend over, side by side, over the back of the Victorian sofa in the drawing room.

We had been bickering all day because Mandy wanted to go to Paris for the weekend and I didn't. I loathe Paris, but neither did I want to let them go away together and strengthen the relationship from which I was being slowly excluded. Mandy minced into the drawing room, preceded by his cologne. He had been at the tongs and had made his long black hair into Farrah Fawcett flick-ups. His feet were bare and his toenails had been painted red.

I was curled up in Daddy's lap in his armchair. He was putting a plaster on my finger and whispering to me. I wanted to stay there for ever, warm and close to him, enveloped in love and safety. I was wearing a tight pink Aertex shirt, which was far too small for me, a pleated black leather miniskirt, ankle socks and shiny black patent-leather Mary Jane shoes with adorable gold buckles.

I was completely happy and so was Daddy, but when Mandy arrived, so did a whining high-pitched voice and all the tension that an unpleasant personality inevitably brings to any atmosphere.

He went over to the drinks tray, poured himself a crème de menthe, added ice and twirled around on his feet like a ballet dancer, glass in one hand, other hand on hip. He walked towards us as if he was on a catwalk, sipped the green liquid and looked down with an expression last seen on the features of the latter stages of the portrait of Dorian Gray. That is, his mouth and eyes were twisted with uncontrolled and unconcealed loathing.

'What ees wrong with diddy-dums?' Mandy said. 'Hurt her lickle finger?'

If I had been a dog I would have bitten him in the face. As it was I leaped up and pushed him incredibly hard so that he fell over. He knocked over an occasional table and went down with a nineteenth-century Spode vase cast in the colour known as Sardinian green. This was followed by an Hermès ashtray and a lamp bearing a picture of the hunt in full cry. Several seconds stood still as both Daddy and I looked at the sprawling ladyboy covered in shards of broken porcelain. They stood still and they were slow, but we did nothing with them. Mandy, however, had the reflexes of a survivor of the streets. He was young, he had been to the gym, he was lithe and wiry and he had fought in slums. The queer left, the hustler arrived and with the hustler a brutish strength and an instinct to use it that overcame any sense of either personal safety or boundary of the law. The macho myth that he had created for himself was no longer distant and far fetched. I sensed genuine danger as he sprang at me and began to close his fingers around my neck. Daddy dragged him off and, picking him up with surprising strength, threw him over the back of the sofa, pulled down his jeans, and held him there, arse up, face in the cushions. Mandy squirmed and wriggled and swore in Spanish.

'Calm down,' Daddy said.

Mandy was so surprised he was silent.

I was as furious as Mandy, breathing hard and crimson. My hair was all over my face and it would not have taken much for me to burst into tears.

Daddy fixed me with steely guardian stare. 'Go and bend over next to him, Stella.'

I pouted and did nothing.

He grabbed me, took my black cotton pants down to the top of my thigh and slapped me hard on the top of the front of my leg. 'Do as you're told. I am not dragging you over there. You go there yourself.'

I was so angry now I didn't know what to do with myself.

He slapped me again, harder, so that the top of my right leg began to turn red. 'Go and bend over the back of the sofa now. I am going to punish you both.'

I knew I had to go there in the end, so I did as I was told. I walked with as much dignity as I could muster to the Aubusson over which my opponent was bent, bare-arsed naked, breathing hard and muttering in Spanish.

I reached my hand to Mandy's crotch to see if he was hard. He was and, for a fleeting moment, I became excited enough to fuck him. He didn't have a bad dick after all, being smooth and brown and thick. It would have done very nicely, attached, as it was, to a person who fucked for a living.

Daddy pulled my hand away from Mandy and put it behind my back. 'Right,' he said, 'that's it.'

Daddy tied my hands behind my back with his St Laurent tie.

Then he pulled my pants down to the floor. Now Mandy and I were two bottoms in a row; four buttocks, if you like to be precise.

I knew what was coming, of course, but this was the first time somebody had received the infliction with me. The pseudo insults of guardianship, the dealing with naughtiness, the punishing – I had only ever experienced these alone, a drama to be enjoyed by Daddy and me alone. Upset though I was, I was also heightened and enjoying the beginning of this new adventure as I liked all sensual experimentation. Immersing myself into the moment, I wondered who would receive it first. I wondered who would get it harder. I wondered how angry Daddy actually was.

I couldn't see Mandy because my face was in the back of the sofa, but I could feel him and I could certainly smell him.

Daddy's voice came from behind us. 'I have had enough of both of you. You are spoiled and childish and unbearable. If it doesn't stop, one of you will have to go.'

Neither of us said anything. I was enjoying the familiar experience of warm arousal. I hoped that Mandy was taking all this very badly and would walk out.

Daddy left the room for five long minutes and we were left in our mutual hatred, bare bums in the air, waiting and humiliated. I rubbed my throbbing pussy against the back of the sofa. If my hands had not been tied behind my back,

I would have played with myself. I prayed that Daddy would fuck me at the end of this session; the sexual need for him was unbearable.

The only sounds were of the clock and the purr of traffic travelling down the Embankment. I knew that Susan was in the house, downstairs in the kitchen. I wondered if she would appear. I hoped not.

Silence.

Who would Daddy beat first, and would there be any significance in his choice? I heard Daddy come back into the room and his shoes pad across the carpet. He spanked me first and he used a leather-backed paddle. I screamed the place down. I screamed out the pain of the present, the frustration of the near past and, then, without any inhibition at all, I shouted out the pain of the past. I had never let rip like this; it was a new surrender and I lost myself into it, the release and the smacking, the throbbing, the blood, the trust in Daddy.

Mandy was undoubtedly alarmed, thinking that the noise I was making related to the levels of pain being meted. This was not quite true. I was yelling because I needed to yell, as a baby sometimes does, just because there is unbearable and unfathomable frustration about which there is nothing one can do. Daddy was hurting me, yes, but if he had been hurting me in a real relation to the fuss I was making he would have been removing my leg with a pair of nail scissors.

Mandy was a drama queen and should have been able to perceive that I was making an unnecessary fuss, but he was also ego-centred, blind with narcissism and could not read other people with any accuracy. He probably thought he was about to receive an unbearable punishment.

Daddy had used the paddle on me before. Once I had received it after throwing a fork at him; another time he caught me smoking a joint out of the window. The paddle allowed him to judge the punishment from the colour of my buttocks. Sometimes he would go for a light pink shade, into red, crimson and then purple. Today was the darker shade of that spectrum.

He spanked me really hard, stopping in between so that I knew he was planning to go on. This was a proper punishment and, for the first time for some time, it brought the desire for behaviour change. He was telling me that if I didn't conform to his desires, I was going to lose him.

I did cry.

Daddy pulled me up into a standing position, pulled me towards him and untied my hands. He knelt down and pushed his tongue into my wet cunt. I came instantly, shuddering and violent. I fell. He caught me and kissed me on the mouth. Then he told me to be quiet and watch. I stood there, naked from the waist down, three fingers in myself, my bottom throbbing with red heat. I hardly knew where I was.

He then meted out the same punishment on Mandy's smooth brown backside and that backside danced a merry dance, jiggling to escape the unforgiving leather, growing pinker as Mandy became angrier and angrier and harder and harder. Mandy had to be spanked for more than fifteen minutes before he showed any sign of genuine remorse. He was not a natural submissive, he was merely undergoing this rite in order to maintain his position with a necessary source of money. Eventually, as Daddy continued to rhythmically tan that backside, the cursing subsided and Mandy became silent.

'Are you going to behave yourself?'

'*Si*,'

'Yes what?'

'*Si, señor.*'

Mandy stood up, rubbed his arse and scowled.

Daddy did not kiss him. No aftercare for Mandy. Served him right.

'Stand there, Mandy, please,' said Daddy.

Daddy pushed me down on all fours onto the carpet in front of the fireguard. Kneeling behind me he inserted his hard dick deep into me, his pelvis crunching against my flaming red buttocks. I was in another space, transported by pain and pleasure, everything hot, my throat open, groaning my need for him.

He did me slowly. It was delicious. He ejaculated into me, taking long minutes to relish his orgasm. Then he stood up, pulled his trousers up and said to Mandy, 'Tell Stella that she is beautiful.'

I remained on all fours, knowing that if I sat on the floor it would hurt my arse.

'Tell her.'

Mandy looked as if he was about to cough up a hairball. But his arse was sore and he didn't want any more. He knew that he had to do as he was told. 'She is beautiful.'

After that we both had to clear up the mess we had made during the fight. Daddy gave us dustpans and brushes and told us that we had destroyed five thousand pounds worth of china.

We were slightly subdued. I knew Mandy wanted to talk, to gain some mutual bonding from the pain, some mutiny against the authority figure. But I didn't want to be friends. Cruel and kind. This was Daddy's métier – his art form. He was affectionate to me but he remained obsessed with Mandy.

I learned to be patient. I learned to watch as if I were an audience waiting for the narrative lines to play out. I had read enough Buddhism to understand the sense in detaching from outcome. It was right. I knew I had to let go, but I did not disconnect from what I wanted. I wasn't that Buddhist!

Daddy meanwhile was selling shares. I heard one of his (only) close friends tell him off about it in the drawing room. Rodney said that Daddy was making a fool of himself, though he didn't call him Daddy of course. He admonished him about the girl bride (which I assume was me) and the screaming poof (Mandy seemed to be the only candidate for this description). Rodney told him that he was ruining his reputation, undermining his business interests and mismanaging his portfolio. He was allowing two little gold-diggers to bring him down.

I couldn't hear Daddy's response because his voice was too low and I refused to put my ear to the keyhole like a pantomime butler.

China and silver continued to disappear from the house. Daddy blamed Jimmy and Susan who had worked for him for years. This, unsurprisingly, caused a rift. Jimmy might have 'previous for grevious' (as he put it) but he had neither stolen from his employer nor intended to do so. He was a changed man, he told me in the shrubs; he had turned his life around through AA. If all this carried on he would have to leave.

'It's goin' to end up me or that Spanish tealeaf,' he told me.

I told Jimmy to be patient. I was working on it.

'I'll take it by the day,' he said gloomily. 'One day at a time. Keep it simple. Let go. Let God.'

There was bound to be a final scene and there was. The three of us had had a tense dinner in Park Walk when I saw Mandy steal the tip that had been left by another table. He forced it into the hip pocket of his tight jeans, where it sat as a rectangular protuberance of evidence.

When we returned to Cheyne Walk, I told Daddy what I had seen. I also told him that Kevin the hairdresser had seen Mandy pulled over by the police for soliciting in Earl's Court.

'That is a lie!' Mandy shrieked.

Daddy, to my surprise, believed me. He didn't seem to mind the soliciting but he was furious about the tip. I knew why. If Mandy had been seen, Daddy, as a regular customer, would have been held accountable and seen as ridiculous. In his view, stealing a tip from a waiter was unforgivable, especially when the thief had everything he needed and a great deal more.

Mandy could have denied it and got away with it, but, stupid as he was, in the way criminals often are, he admitted to this infraction and said so what.

'They are all reech cunts.'

'The waiters aren't rich,' I pointed out.

'Ssh, Stella,' said Daddy. 'Mandy, I want you to give me that money. I will go tomorrow and tip the waiter.'

'You out your tiny mind? Nowayman.'

Daddy and I stared at the note sticking from his hip pocket.

'I mean it, Mandy. I want the money you stole from that table.'

'*En el nom de Dio!* Ees five pounds!'

I did not know whether he meant that this was a lot (too much to give back) or too little to worry about. I suppose five pounds is like beauty, subject to the eye of the beholder. I didn't know about tips; Daddy always did all that. I never even asked.

'I don't care, give it to me.'

I had never seen Daddy this cold and determined. Suddenly, he was the professional businessman, dealing in the boardroom, cool and clever. He would not be manipulated or conned and he was going to get exactly what he wanted.

'You go fuck yoself motherfucker,' said Mandy.

Mandy's perceptions were limited. If he had read this scene with accuracy, he would have seen that this was the moment to apologise and do as he was told. Not only was he stupid, but he was accustomed to Daddy's dependence. He had never seen a strong side of him, only the older lover who always tried to please him.

'I want you to leave,' said Daddy.

If you have ever been unfortunate enough to witness violence you will know that it is mundane. It does not arrive with music. There are no Asian policemen. We were in the kitchen. Daddy was standing by the fridge. Mandy pulled a knife and lunged at him. He drew back his hand and stuck it in as hard as he could. Daddy crumpled to the ground with a moan. Blood spattered onto the fridge and a sticky red pool began to ooze onto the floor.

Mandy did not look shocked and he did not run. He stood calmly surveying his result, carefully tore off a square of kitchen roll, wiped the knife on it and put the stained sheet into the bin. Then he slowly walked out of the room, his Cuban heels clacking up the wooden stairs and into the distance.

I rang an ambulance.

8. 1986–7

The wound was only in the leg as it turned out. Painful. Some loss of blood. Not lethal. Daddy was confined to a wheelchair. It had brakes but I didn't know where they were. I pushed him around the place so fast that his hair took on a windswept look.

'Stella, this is not a toy, mind that woman. Christ.'

My biceps became muscular and toned.

A private nurse came every day to check his dressing and ensure he had enough painkillers. She would scrutinise me with undisguised suspicion as I pranced around Daddy's sickroom in short skirt, knee-high socks and a tight T-shirt portraying the face of the very wonderful Tom Verlaine.

'Your daughter has a lot of energy, sir. But they do when they're young. I remember the days when I could shimmy 'til way past midnight. Now I'm in bed with a cup of cocoa and the cat.'

'She is not my daughter!' Daddy said with as much strength as he could muster. 'Stella, stop dancing about like that, you'll knock something over. Get away from that escritoire. Go and get Nurse Grey a cup of tea.'

'That would be lovely, dear.'

I clumped off in the lace-up Viv Westwood's and returned with the requested refreshments having eaten most of the chocolate biscuits myself and leaving the boring ones for the nurse. I didn't trust Nurse Grey. She was of an age. Forty-eight at least, she could wheedle her way into Daddy's weakened affections and prolong his illness for her own ends. I didn't read the newspapers, but I suspected that kind of thing was in them. Daddy had mentioned that he would like a nurse, after all. After the Mandy incident I was on my guard against any form of intervention. There were to be no more ménages.

'Lovely china.'

'Yes. She has used the Seuter coffee pot for some reason,' he said glaring at me. 'It's worth five thousand pounds.'

'I don't think we should smoke in the sick room, do you, dear?'

'Stella, put that cigarette out at once!'

We spent hours in his bed talking and stroking and not doing anything much. I would give him slow blow jobs and he would bring me to orgasm with his fingers, telling me how he was going to fuck me soon, that I was a bad girl, that his dick was going to go up my arse, my bad girl's dirty arsehole. I was his own girl and I was going to as I was told.

I would spread my legs and take it, his hard dick in me, his big hard cock. I would whine and say I wanted it now, I wanted my Daddy's dick in me, but we both knew I couldn't have it. Not yet. We whispered love and hate to each other, all the dirty dialogues of those intense moments, the weird drama of passion when we could both be exactly who we wanted to be, ids unleashed.

Sometimes I danced for him. I would start off in baby-doll pyjamas and my ostrich-feather mules from Frederick's of Hollywood. Daddy had bought them for me, of course, being a perv.

I would draw the heavy damask curtains and turn the lights off as he sat up on his mountain of Egyptian cotton pillows, an alert audience and ready for me. There was a fire in the grate and candles flickered from silver candelabras on his antique dressing table, all enhanced by the pier gilt mirrors.

Slowly, coltish legs on mules, tottering a little at first as I decided on my choreography, I would find my style. Inspired by burlesque, perhaps, rather than the lewd lap dancing of Manhattan, I managed to incorporate the sensuality of strip with a Japanese schoolgirl ethos – that is, I could strip for Daddy in a way that was half girl taking her pyjamas off and getting into bed and half punk with a lean white body and a tattoo on her cunt.

I danced naked for him, wiggling my pert little cheeks in front of his face, rotating my pelvis lewdly so that he could see my minge, smell it, want it, then I would flick away again, twirling in the distance, a nude white figure, slim hips, slim legs, round white breasts, brown nipples.

I was good at creating private entertainment. I hope I still am. I learned that art from my gay friends. It cheered Daddy up to see me perform for him, his own private show, when he was weak and bored. I suppose I was the slave entertaining the sultan, doing what women have always done for their men, terpsichorean foreplay!

He felt his demoralised dick strengthen and, though he couldn't fuck me for some time, because of the wound, I like to think that I contributed to the recovery of his health. I made him watch *Carry On* films and he made me watch cricket. We had the television at the end of the bed.

Privately I was frustrated by his invalidity; he had lost control and was vulnerable, no longer the superior protector, but a convalescent who tired easily and was obsessive about the timing and amount of his medications.

I can only assume that patients are called that because they try it. If I had been born with a maternal instinct, his helplessness might have inspired unconditional affection, but it did not, it annoyed me and, on some days, frightened me. I began to realise that I depended on him.

I tried not to allow my baser defects to subsume good intentions and did my best to be his friend in this hour of need when he was brought down not only by a nasty injury but by the knowledge that Mandy had made a fool of him. His judgement had been wrong; he knew that and it disorientated him.

The police never found Mandy. We all assumed that he had left on one of his fake passports. Daddy was nervous that he would return and he became concerned about security. He employed a man called Stan, a friend of Jimmy's. He had once been a policeman but they had shared a cell in HMP Leyhill. I never found out what Stanley had done, but Jimmy told me that he was 'on the programme'. By this he meant that Stanley attended AA meetings. Stan was about sixty and didn't look tall enough to have been a policeman but he knew a lot about CCTV.

He put in cameras and television screens and the best alarm system money could buy. There were panic buttons and nobody could enter without being seen first. So, of course, I stood at the front door with my top off to amuse Daddy, who could see my brazen tits on the black-and-white image on a screen.

'Do not do that,' he said. 'Stan will see you mucking about. And for God's sake put your top on, this is not a brothel.'

'I thought you liked my tits.'

'I do, but I don't wish the street to see them, thank you.'

I did not think that Mandy would return but my reasoning had not been undermined by a knife in the leg.

'Do you think you will fall for other men?' I asked Daddy.

'Who knows? I am susceptible to beauty as we both know. I get carried away. I want to buy it and possess it.'

'Perhaps you should stick to antiques,' I said. 'Safer.'

'Perhaps you're right. Perhaps I should spend more time taking you in hand. Bend over and lube yourself. I want you.'

'What about the injury?'

'I'll cope.'

'Nurse Grey will be cross if you break your stitches.'

'Be quiet.'

I lay naked with my back to him and in his arms. Slowly, carefully, he lubed his hard dick and pushed it into my rectum where it stayed without movement and I felt, not for the first time, that I was totally in the possession of an insurmountable higher power, an all-subsuming energy that was deep deep inside me. I relaxed; he did not pump, or thrust, or engage in any energetic actions. His dick stayed hard in me, still and silent, allowing me to feel the full sensation of it in me. Then, slowly, he moved his pelvis, easing himself gently in and out, and I was so young and defenceless and in love and vulnerable. He buggered me like that for a long time, and I went to places that were not of the bedroom, that were hardly me, old places, but with no detail. His hands were on the back of my neck, my hair; his lips were on my neck. He came.

'I love you, my Stella,' he whispered close to my ear. 'Don't leave me.'

Tears came to my eyes. He needed me. This confused me. Nobody had ever needed me before and this incited a range of rebellious reactions whose effects were to confuse and upset. I did not know what they meant. I had kept things so simple, and now they were becoming complicated. Real. What were the responsibilities of being needed? What would I actually have to do? Where would my youth go? Was he asking me to leave the cocoon of fabulous Lolita-hood and emerge as a fully-fledged Chelsea housewife? I didn't want him to need me and I didn't want to need him. It felt frightening and asphyxiating. It felt as if a rock had been removed and now all predators could see me and bite my head off. It felt dangerous without being exciting. I realised that I was an emotional coward – that I had thought I was brave because I engaged in daring sexual adventures, brooked no limits, gambled with my sex soul without caring too much about either the stakes or the results. All I wanted was to know more, but only about sensuality. Not about reality. Reality was of no interest to me, no interest to me at all. And I thought I was interested in truth, but I wasn't really. I was interested in fantasy and escape and recycling personal delusion. Daddy's neediness, his new reality, began to bring these to the fore of my inner life where they lingered, begging to be addressed and refusing to move.

'Do you think I should have therapy?' I said to him during this time.

'Don't be absurd,' he said.

Daddy could not understand why he had allowed a dangerous element into his life and what could I say? Nobody knows the answers to the mysteries of the human emotions; there can only ever be interesting theories and ideas whose validity relies on the resonance of experience rather than the logic of scientific breakthrough. I would find him lying in bed, varifocals and *Telegraph*s all over the silk cover, staring through the white chink of light that streaked through the heavy bedroom curtains. He would be immersed in thought and silenced by sadness and I knew he had been wounded inside as well as out.

'I can't believe I could have been so stupid.'

'We're all stupid.'

'God. I went to nightclubs. I'm fifty-three years old. Why didn't I see it coming? Everyone else did. Rodney warned me months ago. Why didn't you say anything? And I think he took one of the Sevres vases; it was worth ten thousand pounds for crying out loud.'

I gawped. Say anything!? It was obvious I loathed the man. What did he want me to say?

'Surely the scene in the restaurant must have told you something,' I replied. 'I hated him on sight. I hated him the first moment I walked into the house and saw that white pochette thing he carried around on his wrist. And smelled him. Christ! I knew he was a liar and thief. I told you that Kevin said he blew up that man's yacht. I did tell you!'

'I thought you were jealous and trying to get rid of him. You have to admit you are prone to exaggerate. Petty theft, yes, a prison sentence, yes, but not some scene out of *Miami Vice*. I know where he came from, remember, and Caracas is no picnic ground.

'He was so different with me once we were alone. He wasn't always as you saw him. He had a sweet nature really ... don't look at me like that, Stella, he did. When I first met him he was a waiter, but there were sisters and brothers starving to death. He couldn't make it on the tips so he started going home with the clients. He was pretty and innocent then. He comes from a place where money is survival, and you do everything you can to get it. He became contaminated by the people who bought him, rich and cruel and stupid. So by the time he came here he was more like them.

'I just couldn't stop myself fancying him; I just couldn't. And because I didn't want to stop myself, I refused to believe the stories about him, especially when they came from Kevin the hairdresser.

'I thought Mandy was a little wayward and, as you know, I like wayward as a personality characteristic. God knows I've had to deal with you.'

'I am not and never will be the same as that man,' I pointed out. 'I am not dishonest or greedy. I am not spoiled. I do not like making people unhappy. And I am far far better dressed than he could ever hope to have been.'

I flashed the egg-shaped fake diamond that I had taken to wearing on my engagement finger. My nails were neither long nor painted as Daddy did not allow it. He liked my nails to be short and my hands to be washed when he told me to wash them, before meals and so on.

'Take that thing off, nobody is going to think you're engaged. It's patently from Butler and Wilson.'

'Kevin thought it was real. I've told him you have connections with De Beers after all.'

'I think we have convincingly established that Kevin is unskilled in key areas of the deductive processes.'

'Nonsense. He is a very good dancer – much better than you – and he is a wonderful hairdresser.'

'His own hair does not advertise either of those facts,' Daddy said not for the first time. He objected to Kevin's hair on the grounds that it was yellow and moulded into a quiff.

This was an homage to Billy Idol, which was perfectly acceptable in my view, but Daddy condemned Kevin on the grounds of this style.

'Kevin does my hair,' I reminded him. 'And I always look lovely, as I think you will agree. There's nothing he can't do with a Louise Brooks bob.'

Daddy brushed my face with his finger. 'You always look lovely. Are you my good little girl?'

'No, I'm not.'

He smiled. 'We'll have a nice time when I am better,' he said. 'Perhaps we'll go away.'

We relaxed. We had to. And though there were many moments of physical comfort and safe companionship, and laughing, there were also times when I felt my chest tighten and a scream build in my throat. I got headaches. I longed to escape and run or fly around the globe or walk across fields or swim in seas. Escape. Escape. Escape. I did the washing-up and made him meals on trays and played board games with him. I drew a line at the crossword puzzle and he drew a line at Cluedo.

'You can't play with two.'

'Jimmy might join in.'

'It's not appropriate. Be quiet. I need to sleep.'

'Can I watch a *Star Wars* video?'

'No.'

I was so good. But sometimes I just couldn't help myself and felt compelled to irritate him to get a reaction. I would complain and whine. It's amazing he never lost his temper.

'Stella, you're bored, go out and play,' he would say.

'I don't want to.'

'Do as I say. Go and play and I'll see you tomorrow.'

'Can I have the credit card?'

'No.'

'But.'

'No, Stella. Don't argue.'

'Can I have a dog?'

'No. We've talked about this. You can have a rabbit.'

'I don't want a rabbit, I want a dog. Why can't I have one of those puppies in Harrods?'

Daddy sighed. 'I'll think about it.'

'Hooray!'

'You'll be wanting to have a baby next,' he said, having the last word and causing me to run screaming from the room.

I thought about taking the credit card and buying a puppy anyway but that would have been stealing and who wanted to be like Mandy? I suspected that if I brought a puppy back to Cheyne Walk I would have been allowed to keep it, but I didn't want to hurt Daddy or take advantage of him. He needed me to be sensible and I did my best to be so.

I would descend to some basement club with my friends or see a goth band or buy books or potter around in my flat scribbling in my diaries and trying to work everything out.

Daddy rarely analysed human behaviour or emotions. He could do cryptic word puzzles and remember long boring verses written by Tennyson, or how much a rectory had cost in Chalfont St Giles in 1978, but he could not address the political complexities of gender relations. Nor did he wish to. I suspect he did not dare to look at it closely in case he found something in himself that he did not wish to see. He always changed the subject if I embarked on his need to father me.

'It isn't sexy to talk about it,' he would say. 'Just as it is not sexy to look at a nipple through a microscope. Sex cannot be erotic without an element of mystery. Eat your ice cream.'

So I was left to draw my conclusions alone.

I thought a lot about submission and how it was central to the process of successful reproduction. The courtships of nature are feathers and frenzy, but, mantis aside, the female must accept the man, and remain still and sublime in order to receive his genes. In the 1980s provocative and clear-thinking feminist writers described the relationship between transgression and self-realisation. Like many ideologies, pure feminism denied the instincts. As communism was flawed by its denial of human greed, feminist thought asked the woman to deny her true nature and did not take into account either the sexuality of biological fact, or the history of messages advertising aesthetic ideals. It is unsurprising that most of the dogma arrived from the lesbian ghetto, where women were less likely to need men or babies and more likely to accept an alternative beauty.

What could I do? I liked sex and wished to have it; I did not have any desire to breed, but there was still a problem. I had to receive. I was supposed to be pursuing an ideology of independence but in order to enjoy recreational sex I had to submit.

Sometimes I wondered if the anti-porn pro-life brigade were right and it was all about rape; if, knowing that I had no control over the force and urge of male strength, I had set up a system of controls that allowed me to be violated under the appearance of my own consent. Certainly I felt that penetrative sex invaded an essential privacy, that the nerve endings of the womb linked with places of inexplicable emotion and forgotten history and there was a conscious need to protect them. I wondered if introducing complex and controllable drama was a way for the conscious mind to allow essential violation.

I knew one thing for sure.

It wasn't simple.

I did not talk about these things with Daddy. The nymphet is a muse – she does not speak, or make sense, she must provoke and entice, incite and inspire. Daddy didn't want a bluestocking, he wanted a white ankle sock. I knew that. I didn't mind particularly, though I wished that he could be the fount of all knowledge and tell me true and wise things, which would help me develop a useful philosophical framework from which to organise my life.

When he offered no answers, my confusion caused me to separate myself from him. I wanted him to know everything – I didn't want to have to work things out for myself; I wanted to be told. I wanted to know what was right and what was wrong. Why did I want a daddy? Because I didn't have one? Because, at heart, most women feel abandoned at some level, because even the lucky ones with good daddies have to suffer a separation? Because I was in touch with my sensibilities and unafraid to play out what I wanted? Because I was stunted and mad and masochistic and he was a nonce?

I did not know if there were other women enacting these scenarios. I felt alone in our age play, but neither did I think I was unique in desiring it. There were few intimations that I represented any form of universality – to look at the women of the 1980s who had left their girlhood well behind in order to carry the shoulders of Alexis Carrington power. Ah. But to look at the women of now? Of the early twenty-first century? They have made their bodies into those of 10-year-old children – huge thyroid eyes, no hips, no tits, Belsen biceps. They have made themselves prepubescent. What are they saying with their rexy stance? They are saying, because I can't handle the real power that has been won for me by real women I am retaining power over my body. I have it all but I have nothing. I am a little girl. I wear little girl's sizes bought in little girls' shops. Look after me. I am too young to get a job; my body can't have children and I am too young to fuck. It's a far cry from my youth when we were too drunk to fuck.

Daddy allowed me to be anything I wanted. He allowed me to act out the old anger and confusion, and he punished me enough to release it. I lost myself in pain and performance and, by so doing, found myself again. I could be spontaneous and that spontaneity charged my sexuality.

*　*　*

By the time Mandy left, I was in my late twenties, leaning towards thirty, though I did not dare to think about it, thirty being an unacceptable age by any stretch of the imagination. I dreaded having to be a thirty-year-old person. They were parents and teachers! Would I have to stop wearing girly hairstyles? Would I have to get some sort of a job?

Some of my friends were beginning to get proper jobs and even be a success. I wondered if I should get a job, but could not imagine what that job would be. None of the Black family had jobs, being unemployable, rich and half cut.

There was no culture of gainful employment, no work ethic in the Black gene pool. The few relations I had come across, spent their days racing or attending to the ever-dwindling pockets of land, which they sold to pay for the racing. The rest stood by the fireplace wearing corduroys. Some of them also made fences in their fields. The women, being beautiful, had married well and spawned.

It could be said that their existence was pointless, but I had always thought that existence was pointless whether you had a job or not. Life was many hours to fill in before you died; a lucky few made contributions that mattered – towards medical breakthrough, or saving lives, but I wasn't ever going to be qualified to do anything of genuine importance. I accepted that and I did not mind, but neither did it drive me towards the job centre.

I still wanted my daddy but his convalescence under-mined the fantasy and began to reveal chinks of reality. They were unwelcome but they were arriving and had to be accepted. I was beginning to see things.

I preferred a role player to the intimacy that is supposed to arrive with so-called mature relationships. I did not know what intimacy was; I assumed that it related to some domestic scenario involving a resilient attitude to smells and fluids and character defects. I suspected that laundry was involved.

I had allowed Daddy to see an important part of me and I made myself more vulnerable to him than many people do. I was his child after all; I opened up that part of myself, and that part could have been easily abused by cruelty.

I wondered whether the roles we had created to communicate with each other had been so successful that we had turned into them. That, for five years, I had remained stunted in my own choice; by finding a daddy, I had stayed where I was, and had developed in a different way. I was an actress who could not walk away from the character she had created for herself, a character in which she was comfortable but which also, in some ways, incarcerated her.

I thought about this but I didn't worry too much about it. I never worried about anything that much, having learned at a young age how little power one can exert over circumstances and people. Perhaps I was too passive, certainly I was lazy. I preferred to be Daddy's girl than make any effort to walk out into the ghastly world of yuppies and perms and City boys celebrating themselves. I was safe in Daddy sanctuary and quite willing to stay there, warm and cosy with a smacked bottom and a full cunt.

The Thatcher economy bred a culture of money as a symbol of success, but my milieu was bohemian and self-indulgent and did not fall in with the ideas of the zeitgeist. I had no need to prove myself or to expose myself on a public stage in order to feel validated. I did not even want to be on television, which, in itself was unusual. Everyone wanted to be on television, even intelligent people wanted to be on television without realising that they would look absurd. I mean, have you ever seen anyone from television in real life? They are all short, orange and sinister. The only question is whether they were short, orange and sinister before they got onto television, or whether there is a biochemical process whereby being on television produces those characteristics? Something to do with the lights perhaps.

Daddy never asked me if I intended to pursue gainful employment and when I brought the subject up he tended to argue against it. I suspected (in my darker moments) that he wanted to retain control. I began to suspect that in that old-fashioned Victorian dad there actually was a Victorian dad, that there was some kind of double bluff going on. 'Of course women should work, if they want to, if they have to. They have as much right to do that as anyone else. But I have not noticed that it has made them happier,' he said smugly. 'The first excuse they get they run off, have babies and expect the man to pay for it all.'

'I might want to get a job one day,' I suggested.

'Why would you want to do that? You don't need the money.'

'I don't know. Because everyone else does?'

'I hadn't put you down as wanting to run with the herd.'

This was true.

'Anyway what would you do?'

'I've got a degree – I could teach.'

He would snigger in a slightly unpleasant way and return to his Dick Francis novel.

My friend Conrad opposed this view. He was always telling me off for being a layabout. I had known him for years. He had lived near us in the country and his parents had occasionally taken me in when my grandmother disappeared or, on one occasion, was taken away.

He had become a successful investigative journalist and had made his reputation by being annoying to Sinn Fein. Conrad was respected and well known. He had even appeared on television without turning orange.

He had done something with his life and couldn't understand why I chose to do so little.

'You're bright and brave,' he said one evening while we were drinking a bottle of wine in my flat. 'Why aren't you doing anything useful?'

'I've had a tattoo on my cunt – a scorpion.'

I wanted to show it to him and I knew him well enough to know that he wanted to see it – who wouldn't? – but he feigned a statesmanlike maturity.

'Good for you,' he said. 'You must be very proud. What else have you been doing?'

'Getting laid.'

'That's a full-time job, is it?' He looked at me with his big honest brown eyes.

'God, you're bossy,' I retorted. 'Yes, it is now you mention it.'

'How's your grandmother?'

'I don't know – she was fabulously rude to me when I rang up and we haven't spoken since.'

'When was that?

'Two years ago.'

He breathed out and assumed an expression of resigned amazement. 'You Blacks,' he said.

'What do you mean?'

'Well.'

' "Well" what?'

He wouldn't enlarge and I sensed truths so terrible that even Conrad could not tell them. Fortunately for my mental equilibrium he wasn't around much, being engaged in dangerous undercover work of a useful and revelatory nature.

One day I turned up at Cheyne Walk and it was clear that Daddy was feeling much better.

'Your make-up is smudged. You look like a trollop.'
'Not Joanna I hope.'
'Don't answer back.'

I was wearing shorts, so it must have been summer. Shorts and a ripped T-shirt, as I recall, with a neat little pair of Patrick Cox tie-up canvas ankle-boots in tan and brown. Daddy and I had seen them in a window in Sloane Street when I was pushing his wheelchair around.

'Go and have a bath and don't come back into this room until you're clean.' He was definitely getting better. 'Who did you play with? Rough boys?'

I hadn't as it happened. The boys of my age were far from rough. They wore lipstick and did art. They were limp and lovely and couldn't have opened a bottle of wine without straining something. They chose great cars but were unable to mend them. They wore dresses and Doc Martens and knew the date of Poe's death. God knows where I got them from. If they disappeared it was to go on a road trip in America or hang out in Berlin. We all read *Less than Zero* and agreed with it. Everyone took Polaroids of each other and the cool people had seen *Liquid Sky* and knew Lydia Lunch.

'I haven't been playing with anyone,' I said. 'I've been playing with myself. Anyway. If anyone plays with rough boys it's you!'

There was no answer to that. It was 4 p.m. and I had come round for tea expecting a kiss and a cake. He was out of bed and rolling around the drawing room in his wheelchair. 'You can have your tea, then go upstairs, have a bath, clean that muck off your face and come back down here.'

We had tea. I was slightly flushed and growing wet. I rubbed myself.

'Stop that, Stella. Go upstairs!'

I returned to him clean. Clean face, clean fanny, clean everything. I was naked underneath his navy-blue St Laurent bathrobe.

He was in his dressing gown and pyjamas, in the wheelchair, by the fire, which was lit though the evening was not cold. The drawing room was two rooms knocked into each other. It had a cream carpet, high heavy silk curtains in gold and yellow, striped wallpaper, occasional tables on which there were lamps whose shades were actually trimmed with bobbles.

In one corner there was an effigy of a black man with a gold turban holding up a gold tray. You see them around, these gaudy slaves, I don't know their antique history and do not wish to. I merely recall disliking it as much as I disliked his elephant foot umbrella stand, which he had inherited and for which he had never apologised. My politics, such as they were, were liberal bordering on libertarian. They had been moulded by The Clash, Frank-N-Furter and footage of the liberation of the concentration camps. In my view Daddy did not ask enough questions. We did not talk about these things. Perhaps we should have done. I once pissed punkishly into the elephant foot umbrella stand and he thrashed my arse so that I had to sit on a cushion for a week, the fabric itching my bare red cheeks and causing a prolonged and intense state of arousal with which he played as he pleased. I don't know if it could have been seen as successful in terms of a direct-action protest, but the horrible umbrella stand was relegated to storage.

'Come here.'

I walked towards him.

'Stand in front of me.'

I stood in front of him and he pulled the robe off so that I was naked.

'God, you're beautiful.' He placed his hand between my legs. 'You've trimmed your bush.'

'Yes.'

'I can see the tattoo, which you went and got without my permission.'

I had forgotten about the scorpion on my pubic bone. 'It's nice isn't it?'

'No.'

'Everyone else likes it,'

'What do you mean "everyone else". Who else has seen it?'

'Kevin the hairdresser has seen it, and I showed it to Mr Patel in the tobacconist. He took a Polaroid.'

I didn't tell Daddy about the goth-fuck Stephen. I couldn't be bothered to explain. And, unlike some men, he was not aroused by his own sexual jealousy. I might have wound him up about the subject of Stephen, for my own entertainment, if he had not been nearly stabbed to death. There is only so much a man can take. I enjoyed the fact that Daddy did not want me to see other men; it felt safe.

He managed to convey monogamy without suffocating my spirit, which is a subtle achievement. I do not know whether this was conscious or not; probably not. He did not think about what he was doing in any great detail, unless it was the detailed choreography of one of our scenes.

The tattoo scorpion reminded us both of a period when the distance had been great between us, so great that we had nearly lost each other. The scorpion was not his brand, it defied his possession. This was no bad thing, but it had the desired effect, which was to irritate him.

He pinched the scorpion with two fingers quite hard so that I yelped.

'Bend over in front of me. I want to examine you.'

I pushed my arse towards his lap and touched my toes. He licked his finger and inserted it slowly into my rectum.

I put my hand on my fanny and three fingers in; I was wet immediately.

'I'm cross with you, Stella.'

'I know, Daddy.'

'And not just because of Mr Patel, who should know better. Turn around.'

I stood up and looked down at him. He looked up at me. He was in a wheelchair, but he was a presence, and he was capable of getting out of it, so I did not feel that he was vulnerable, but strong and cross. I knew I was going to get it. And, just as good, I was going to get fucked.

'Are you going to fuck me?'

He indicated his lap. He had put on a pair of leather gloves. So there he was, Brooks Brothers pyjamas, silk dressing gown, slippers, wheelchair, leather gloves. It couldn't have been pervier.

'What about the wound in the leg?'

'Be quiet, Stella, or I will gag you. Make your nipples erect.'

I played with my tits.

He had a hairbrush and he gave me it, ten minutes at least, smacking me into a red blush.

'Ow. No.'

'Yes, Stella.'

Thwap, thwap, thwap, the endless blush of pain and pleasure.

'Let me see your bottom.' He stared at the red-stained peachy crevices and pulled his erect dick out of his pyjamas. 'Now come and sit on me.'

I am flexible and could easily sit astride him in the wheelchair. I smoothed my puss up and down on him, moving my hot arse like a piston, caressing him with my internal muscles, kissing his dick with my cunt control until he shuddered into me.

'Good girl.'
I often wished we had a photo of that.
Stella and Daddy and the motile pervertible.

Soon after this my grandmother died and I had to go back
to Wiltshire.

9. 1987

M y grandmother died in 1987. My return to her house
is described in my diary of that year by the phrases
'RIP Granny' and 'No bananas'. The notes are sometimes
scribbled and cryptic, sometimes alarmingly lucid. 'Bailiffs'
for instance reminds me that they had been and gone and
taken the dining-room table. There is a photograph of
Owen, the wire-haired terrier and caricatures of various
relations so it is possible to describe, with some accuracy,
what happened.

I had to sleep in the bedroom of my childhood, which was
a sinister experience. I had to lie on a single bed on a
withered pale-blue candlewick bedspread and stare at the
fading sweet-pea wallpaper.

There was time to consider the past – those ugly scenes
of solitude and confusion at school. Images floated, unwelcome, across my mind's eye: the hirsute teachers, the
revolting food, the yellow milk; a rat in the downstairs loo;
bad teeth; losing the school uniforms; forgetting the poem;
runny eggs, breaded fish, margarine, being made to sing;

smells that made you retch. And the fear. Fear. Fear. Fear. I had never known where to hide. The large wardrobe, painted in dripping glossy magnolia paint, had creaked of its own volition and was crammed with mutants. Under the bed was out of the question; in the bed, illogically, was safe.

People had felt sorry for me, of course. I was an orphan, after all. So I got away with murder at times. I remember walking away with other children's toys and being allowed to have them. I had no discipline then, ironically. Nobody ever told me what to do; I was unfettered and unboundaried, growing wilder with every year that passed. I was looking for boundaries, I suppose, when I met Daddy, boundaries and love and pleasure.

I remembered the abstract eroticism of childhood; how you don't know at the time but looking back it makes a little more sense, but only a little. I was never touched in either a good or a bad way. Certainly I was never hugged, so I sometimes threw myself at people. Conrad's father used to lift me up and swing me around and make me laugh. So I guess I began to associate physical affection with an adrenalin rush. And I was very much in love with Conrad's father. Conrad later told me that his parents had been genuinely worried about me but that there had been little they could do.

I found a dinky Halcyon Day pot full of my own hair. I had been through a phase of pulling it out, bit by bit, comforted by the compulsion. Little black tufts. Nobody had noticed and I was glad that they had not. Unchecked, I could pull as I pleased. I didn't pull out my hair in order to attraction attention; I pulled out my hair because I had to and would have been irritated if anyone had involved themselves in this all-consuming and satisfying process. I was ten or something.

There was a bookshelf containing every book ever written by Enid Blyton, most of them stolen, as that was the one skill I had, stealing from bookshops. I wanted to knit and play the piano, but neither of these opportunities were offered, so I shoplifted. I needed something to do with my hands, Your Honour.

All Enids were here, all crimes punished, all morals clear, all bottoms reddened by masterful hands. My first porn. My first experience of the wonders of cruelty as evinced in the written word. There is a subculture of sex cartoons called Bondage Fairies – did you know that? Somebody should do a dissertation frankly.

I graduated to the *Beano* and so on, where kids were punished, then to Dickens and Golding and *Black Beauty*, which were as satisfactory for the same reasons, full of awe-inspiring human sadism clearly outlined for those who needed to learn about and accept the full range of cruelties.

A battered doll's house contained forty trolls of differing size and hair colour. There was a teddy about which I cannot think let alone write.

There were small Wellington boots and ballet shoes and exercise books and a ruler from New Zealand. I couldn't help looking at the ruler and wondering if Daddy was missing me.

There were old tubes of hydrocortisone cream, which had been prescribed for the eczema on my face and the spectacles frames (without glass) that I had worn for years as an homage to Brains in *Thunderbirds*.

I had watched television on the black-and-white set in Mrs Erin's sitting room. My grandmother didn't watch television; she listened to the radio and danced with herself. And she read for hours.

I shared the *Dr Who* experience with (the late) Mr Erin who sent the drama of fear up several notches by yelling 'exterminate' whether the Daleks were in the episode or not, his belief being that they were in all episodes. He went even further with these unhelpful theories by saying that the *Dr Who* writer had drawn on real life. The Cybermen, the Yeti and the Ice Warriors were real and secreted in bunkers in London.

This did not decrease the fear-based compulsive obsessive activity in which I was already involved, and I started counting everything in order to prevent being attacked by real robots traveling in from Waterloo station. I counted everything until I went to boarding school and, forced to mix in crowds, the prophecies of Erin faded away.

Wearing the glassless glasses of my childhood, I rummaged through my grandmother's bedroom and, in particular, her medicine cabinet where, as I had both suspected and hoped, there was a mother lode of psycho-pharmaceuticals. The bailiffs had not taken them despite the fact they must have been worth thousands on the street.

I scooped up the clinking brown glass, about a hundred or so bottles, some dating from 1957, and put them in my suitcase where they sustained my spirits as a stash of hope and escape. I was not without suicidal ideation, though it wasn't the actual loss of my grandmother that was inspiring it. I wasn't going to miss her as I had not seen her for the last five years; I was not going to need her because she had never provided security. Raised without expectation, I had never been disappointed. But a gloom descended, a dark all-encompassing cloud of melancholia whose wave was satisfactorily held back by the glorious alchemy of Granny's Drugs. Granny's Drugs – that would be a good name for a band, more 60s than 70s perhaps.

I don't know with what illnesses Granny had been diagnosed, but she had pills to suit every symptom available to the human body – from migraines and shaking leg syndrome to arthritis, insomnia, heart disease and hiccups.

There were analgesics (opioid and non-opioid), ben-
zodiazepines and barbiturates, chloral derivatives and anti-
manics. There was a range of MAO1s and all the pams, as
well as anxiolytics and hypnotics. There were some terrifying uppers in the form of Dexamfetamine and the anti-
psychotic Serenace, which I took first, for the name alone,
and combined with the modified release capsule of hydro-
morphone hydrochloride. I think Mrs Erin thought I was a
little slow as I slumped around in the kitchen, nervous
system in a sedated condition, white wine spritzer in one
hand, cigarette in the other and enjoying a feeling of
unfamiliar optimism.

'I think I am going to be a drug addict,' I said, as if
informing her of my career choice.

'Grief's a funny thing,' she replied. 'Takes different
people in different ways.'

Mrs Erin herself, having sailed through the death of her
husband without a tear, was devastated by the loss of
Granny whom she described, incorrectly, as a 'very good
woman'.

Good at what? I thought. Driving while under the
influence? Playing croquet in the snow? Collecting feathers?
Playing the toy piano? Beating off creditors with an antique
umbrella? Dead-heading roses before they were dead?

Much as I had admired my relation during my early life,
I found that now she had disappeared I was angry, as if she
had at best insulted me and at worst betrayed me.

My 'grief', if that is what it was, took the form of an
ever-increasing resentment about her failings rather than the
nostalgia of respectful affection, which usually colours such
departures.

Mrs Erin, however, sobbed uncontrollably and loudly
into a series of embroidered cotton handkerchiefs, whose
ladylike size was too small to contain the lubrications of

misery. They were rolled up into balls and pushed up in the sleeves of her cardie, where they formed lumpy rows as if her arms had developed a series of tumours.

There had been an oxygen tent apparently and osteoporosis. Nobody had told me. Granny had asked them not to; not, I suspect to spare me, but because she did not wish to be seen in a state of unattractive debilitation.

Mrs Erin had attended the deathbed and said that though 'Mrs B. looked dreadful', she was as 'happy as Larry'. She had wanted to die for quite a long time, and with the arrival of the final release, she was all smiles, is what Mrs Erin said, and I believed her.

Mrs Erin had been left one of the larger piles of cash that Granny had secreted around the house. 'She gave me a note in the hospital, Miss Stella,' she told me. 'Said where to find it. Do you think it's all right, you know with the law?'

'I doubt it,' I said. 'But I don't think that should worry us. The money is yours, Granny meant you to have it and God knows you earned it.'

Mrs Erin had actually saved her life on a number of occasions.

I forgot to ask how much it was, but Mrs Erin spoke of buying a little place in Hove, so I expect it was enough.

'You'll take Owen will you, Miss Stella?'

'Of course,' I said.

'He does bite,' she said, 'though less teeth now, of course.'

'I know,' I said.

'Mr Tremeloe threatened to shoot him.'

'Really?'

'Mrs Forbes's Letitia had to have a tetanus.'

'Blimey.'

'You'll be all right if you don't put your face anywhere near him. He'll have your nose off. And don't pick him up,

Miss Stella, he doesn't like it. Try not to touch him actually, that's probably best.'

It was in a fruitless attempt to oil up to Owen that I took him into the garden. I sat down on the park bench with a can of lager, a couple of diazepam and a Marlboro Light – all habits realising their full potential now that Daddy wasn't around to censure them. Daddy. Where was he? In Hong Kong on business. He had apologised but he had not cancelled.

'Fuck off then,' I had said.

'Don't be silly, Stella. I will only be away for two weeks. Do you want Jimmy to drive you to the station?'

'No.'

He sighed; patient Daddy with recalcritant teenager. 'You had better give me the telephone number of your grand-mother's house.'

'Fuck off.'

We had parted on bad terms.

I began to build a resentment against him, thinking that if he was with me everything would be all right. He would have taken charge. He had experience. He would have hugged me and taken the responsibilities that were too much to bear.

A solicitor drove up the drive in a new black Golf GTI and then stood in front of the fireplace in the drawing room. Young, conscientious and worried, he kept looking at the door to see if someone older and more responsible was going to follow me in.

I was wearing a Bonzo Dog Doo-Dah Band T-shirt and a pair of skin-tight Lycra ski pants with scarlet pixie boots. I had made a badge saying 'Vernon Dudley Bohay-Nowell is God'. I was fond of badges then.

My hair was an array of paper butterflies bought in a stationery shop. They kept falling off and fluttering to the floor, as if dying, in much the same way that Mick had played homage to Brian in Hyde Park.

I was in performance mode and experiencing the paradoxical excitement sometimes inspired by barbiturate abuse. Involved in effect, I was creating and controlling the scenes because this was more pleasant than thinking of dead gran dead as a doornail, dead dad, dead mother, dead parrot, dead everybody. It was easier to think of dead parrots, so I did, and laughed occasionally and at inappropriate moments when the solicitor was explaining things to me.

Mrs Erin had told me that Mrs Black had requested that her body be thrown out in a bin bag and taken away by the rubbish men. The solicitor observed that this was illegal.

Was I sure that Mrs Black was in her right mind when she made her last will and testament?

'No,' I said. 'She did not have a right mind in the conventional sense of the word.'

The solicitor told me that everything had been left to me. This legacy included the house, the land and the debt, whose size, with tax, was equal to the cost of her assets. This meant that, on his calculation, I would walk away with a sum of £59.33.

When the meeting was over, Mrs Erin brought in a tray with tea and biscuits and the young man relaxed slightly, or, at least, he began to speak in a more normal way.

'The thing is, Miss Black,' he said in his ernest Dorset burr, 'it's not a good idea to avoid the Revenue. Are you aware that your grandmother did not fill in anything resembling a government tax form at any point during her life? Or any form at all as far as I can make out. She certainly had no valid driving licence. To be fair, neither did she make any claims on government in the form of pensions and so on, but they don't like it, Miss Black, they don't like it at all. Old ladies with wads of cash hidden about their person is not their thing. They don't think it's funny . . .'

It could have been worse, it could have been a debt that I couldn't pay. But as it was it was evens.

An aunt arrived, a Susan in an Hermès headscarf, unexpected and unwelcome, loving the drama.

'Darling,' she said, 'I've had breast cancer. Now. Who's coming to the funeral? Have you got Lakey and Bill? And what about the Falklands? They'll have to be told. Then there's Denise and Fiona and all those Brownes. And aren't there some cousins in Dubai?'

She looked through her Smythson address book.

'There's Tom and Primmy. Oh no, she's dead. I must cross her out.'

She stalked around to see what she could claim but was battered back by various suits with clipboards who were assessing the probate.

'There's nothing going,' I said. 'Granny left debt.'

'Oh well, Helen was always useless about money, useless. Still that little picture of Cousin Sammy? The frame alone is worth two hundred pounds.'

We went to the funeral parlour. I was quite stoned and the Aunt Susan did all the talking. I brought Owen in an effort to annoy her, but this direct action seriously backfired because rather than bite her, as I had hoped, the dog went after me. Nobody could hear themselves over the growling so I put on a pair of my grandmother's hand-made leather gloves and put him back in the car.

We looked in a catalogue and chose an urn to hold the ashes to ashes and a coffin in which to burn the body, which would have gone up very easily, of course, because of the alcohol.

I let the Aunt choose the music and the flowers. I didn't need this ritual and resented the fact that when it came to the important events of life and death, God was still around the place and nobody argued with Him.

I thought my grandmother was right: the council should have taken her away. It would have been easier and cheaper.

I had no idea who was coming to the service. The telephone was a 50s Bakelite model not dissimilar to the one featured at the bottom of the staircase in *What Ever Happened to Baby Jane*? It rang with a tinny tinkle. I would answer hoping it was Daddy but it was always mad upper-class voices asking if Helen wanted flowers, when she was hardly in a position to want anything.

I would hand the phone to the Aunt who relished her duties and the hushed conversations. 'Yes, she's here. I don't know. I think she's on drugs. It's difficult to tell with the young, isn't it? No, Helen didn't leave her anything, just a bill apparently. No. No, don't worry, I don't think you'll have to stump up for anything.'

Helen Black. Suddenly the shadowy spirits of my childhood started to take on dimensions. In death Granny was becoming a real person. Helen Black, mother of Frank, mother-in-law to Samantha, grandmother of Stella. She had been the mother of my father and so Frank Black too started to turn from an imaginary dad to a real person. The Aunt Susan was my mother's half-sister and I was glad of this, that she was not a whole, because I did not like to think of her being like my mother.

'It's lucky your father made provision for you,' the Aunt Susan said. 'Terrible the way he died. Terrible. And so soon after poor Samantha.'

The Blacks arrived and it wasn't a pretty sight. To my horror, a genetic shape revealed itself – a hereditary adiposity where the women, in middle age, developed barrel stomachs and cabriole legs. There were twenty or so of these fat women. Daddy would have said I was exaggerating and it was probably nearer to three, but it felt like twenty. They all wore mink coats and scarlet lipstick. They were all the same, same coat, same shape, same lips, moving forward as one massive fur ball.

There were also groups of old village sticks who came for a laugh, and several oafs complaining that they were missing the 4.30 at Newmarket.

I wore leather and a veil and a great deal of costume jewellery, which I had found in my grandmother's room after the probate had gone home. Actually it could have been real – some of it was quite heavy and real jewellery often looks fake in my experience. Certainly the Aunt Susan took a break from the proceedings to study it closely, even at one point suggesting that I unhook the pieces so that she could feel them. I wouldn't have trusted the woman to post a letter without steaming the stamp off.

Champagne and salmon sandwiches were served in the drawing room by Mrs Erin and Mrs Forbes's Letitia, the one who had been bitten by Owen.

There were dark squares on the wallpaper where the good pictures had once been and a fire that did not give out enough heat, but a lot of drink, so everyone became inebriated. Tears flowed and tongues flapped. I took some yellow pills, which made me both docile and polite. They were the perfect funeral drug in other words. I received condolences graciously and listened to dreadful information delivered by the unhinged and overfed.

'You're Frank's girl?'

'Yes.'

'She's Frank's girl, Mary, remember Frank, short fella, had a horse? Never won anything, cost a fortune. The horse I mean, not Frank.'

'Oh yes. Frightfully good looking. Rather a good shot when he wasn't pissed.'

'That could be anyone.'

'Liked a young lady as I recall.'

'Who doesn't?'

'Went to Eton with William, same house I think.'

'That's the one.'

'Frank.'

The dead began to walk. Frank Black had arrived. I discovered that he was neither tall nor strong. He wasn't even dark, as I had always imagined. I had received the black sheen from my mother. My father was blond and blue eyed, if you please. Blond and blue eyed and drank in the Green Man pub in Harrods. I had never seen photographs, you see. My grandmother, always in grief, could not see pictures of him and refused to talk about any topic vaguely relating to the issue.

A man in a yellow waistcoat told me that he had been at school with Frank. He had been the shortest man in the year, but also the most anarchic. He was one of the richest boys in the school, monogrammed everything, drank like a fish, first one to own a car (which he hid in the town) and was eventually expelled for going to London and not returning for three days with the excuse that a Jew had bonked him on the head with a shoe and he had lost his memory.

'He was a terrible anti-Semite after that. Still, I suppose everyone was then.'

If I had not been both drunk and sedated, I would have shuddered. As it was, I laughed like a person in an advanced stage of hysteria and heard, not for the first time, the sombre thump of the advancing jackboot.

It all started to come together as the various relatives presented themselves to me.

Frank Black had not gone to university. He had had money. He spent his time going to parties in London and

Paris. He had a lot of friends. He had met Samantha, my mother, on a skiing holiday in Courchevel. They had been in love, but only married for two years, of course, because she had died so quickly. She was 25. He was 26.

'Samantha dying was the end,' one of the more lucid mink coats told me. 'He just couldn't recover. Terribly drunk, poor man. He used to start fights and then lose them because everyone was bigger and stronger than him. He was always being thrown out of places with blood on his collar. He could be very unpleasant when he was drunk – charm personified when sober, but he was never sober. I remember telling him to go to a health farm before he ended up in jail. They are similar, of course – diet wise – but I thought the former was more preferable, if more expensive.

'Then he spent all that money on the race horse, which never won anything. We all thought he had read far too much Ian Fleming. He was living way beyond his means keeping up with that fast set in Gstaad and Cap Ferrat.

'He went bankrupt. Would have gone down completely if your grandmother hadn't bailed him out. There was money there, make no mistake. God knows what Helen did with it, I believe she has left you slightly embarrassed?'

'My father made provision for me,' I said stoutly, wishing to recover some semblance of his memory. 'I have a flat in Chelsea.'

'Oh good. That's a relief. So. What do you think you will do?'

I thought of Granny's stash. 'I think I will do drugs,' I said, 'for a bit.'

'And after that.'

'I might go away.'

'Well,' she concluded, 'it's nice to meet you. Frank never spoke about you, actually. I wasn't even aware he had a daughter.'

The afternoon closed in and late-autumn darkness descended outside. I felt heavy. As if the blood had been sucked out of me. I was climbing the stairs to find an amphetamine when a voice called up. 'I'm here now. You're saved.'

Daddy?

No, Conrad.

His face was raised towards me like a sunflower from the hall in which he was standing, wearing a funeral black overcoat which made him look devastating. Hindsight tells me that this was unintentional. Conrad had no dress sense, it just happened that black overcoats suit everybody.

'Where are you going?'

'Nowhere.'

He climbed up the stairs towards me. I sat down on a step. He sat down beside me.

'How are things going?'

I shrugged. Inept, teenage.

'You look a little glassy eyed. What have they been doing to you?'

'Telling me things I don't want to hear.'

'Bastards,' he said. 'What kind of things?'

I shrugged again. 'Frank Black, my father, not that I care.'

Conrad sighed, put his arm around me, and kissed me on the head.

'Frank Black died when he was twenty-six,' he said. 'He hardly had time to become a person, so try not to care what that lot say. They are not the types to think. Let's face it, most of them look as if they can hardly breathe and speak at the same time.' He pulled a face. 'Dreadful wine. I thought your grandmother had a famous cellar.'

'She drank it.'

'Oh yes. Well. Anyway. Frank Black, your dear father, was about your age when he died, so think about it. He was young. According to my own late beloved father, who knew him quite well, he was a nice man broken by grief. He wasn't too bright. His wife had the brains. She looked rather like you , according to my dad, but I expect you know that.'

Subsumed by an overpowering confusion, disorientation and pure misery, I fell into Conrad.

'Poor little girl,' he said, putting his arms around me. 'You stay here with me.' He smelled wonderful. He was wonderful.

If I had been a normal person, I would have sobbed for the rest of the night. Sobbed and cried and mourned, but I had taken a cocktail of mood-changing substances, so therefore I had no mood that was either identifiable or appropriate to a funereal occasion, except perhaps the occasional bout of genuine amusement.

Conrad followed me up the stairs to my bedroom. I don't think he knew at that moment that we were going to have sex. I think he was just following without thinking, to make sure I was all right.

We had played together as children, but never at my grandmother's house. It had always been at his house, in the garden, and he had always been a little bored with me, being older and wanting to play football. It had only ever worked when one of his parents was around to lead the games or play cards with us. Anyway I never really wanted to play with Conrad, I was only interested in his father.

I lit a candle and we lay side by side on our backs on the candlewick bedspread. It was a lumpy experience due to the age of the mattress and pillows. Most of my make-up was now on my hands which were stained black and purple. I didn't care. It was dark anyway, what did he care?

'Take your coat off, Conrad,' I said.

He did as he was told and then kissed me quite hard on the mouth, hugging me closely to him as he did so.

'This is so wrong,' he said.

'Why?'

'Well. You're completely stoned and grief stricken and I'm taking advantage of you.'

'I thought it was the other way around.'

'That's true.'

He kissed me again. I pushed myself into him, feeling him hard between my thighs.

'Anyway,' I said, 'you've read enough to know that sex and death go together.'

We made love.

He pushed himself slowly into me. Slow and hard, and took his time. I felt every inch of him, wide and thick. He had control. And he was tall, so when he folded me into him I was enveloped and tiny and I love that. I was surrounded by him, melded, and at one – I had never felt this before, not physically. Intellectually, yes, with Daddy, our minds were together, but our bodies? Our bodies were always involved in stage direction. We were close, but not in the same way. Conrad subsumed me without suffocating me and on a deep level I felt his courage and his kindness.

'I can come when I want to,' he whispered quite proudly.

'Well don't,' I suggested, 'I like feeling you inside me.'

We lay together for a long time. I, in his arms, back towards him. He was behind, with his hard warm dick in me, like a dummy in a mouth, I suppose, certainly of great comfort.

'Ah, Stella,' he whispered and moved his pelvis, 'now I must come.'

Gently, he pleased himself, taking me from the back. And I rubbed myself gently at first, and then in time with him. He waited. It must have seemed ages. I came and, as I did so, the vibrations tingling throughout my cunt, he had his beautiful and well-deserved climax.

We dozed. We woke up. I lit a cigarette. He waved the smoke out of his face and said, 'Are you seeing anyone?'

I was coming down.

'Yes.'

'Is it serious?'

'Yes.'

'Long term?'

'Yes. What about you?'

'No. Work. You know. Makes it difficult. I'm about to go to Washington for ages.'

'Oh.'

'So what's he like this chap of yours?'

'Older.'

'Older like Father Christmas, or older like thirty?'

'Fifty-four.'

'Ah-ha.' He looked complacent as if he knew everything. 'Daddy.'

'Yes, Daddy, and I'm not ashamed by the way.'

'I bet he tans your bum and does kinky things with his little girl.'

Conrad was getting another hard-on!

'He does as it happens, not that it is any of your business.'

'I always knew you were naughty and complicated and shameless! You've got it written all over you.'

'You can talk. You're hard.'

I told Conrad about the delicious pain of Daddy's hands beating my flesh until it was red, so that my cheeks, flaming, tingled all day and I couldn't wear pants. I told him how, after these sessions, Daddy would make me wear skirts and would lift them up to look at my behind whenever he felt like it during the day, and we would both be aroused for hours. He would tell me that he needed me to suck him and I would always comply obediently because the memory of the recent punishment was still throbbing through my pelvis and thighs and the nerve endings of all the internal channels.

I told Conrad how Daddy brushed my hair and dressed me and I could sit in his lap for ages, curled up, with my arms around his neck. Or how, having reddened me with a hairbrush, he would make me wait for him. On all fours, flaming arse in the air. Wet, waiting and desperate for him, he would make me wait and, sometimes, he would simply walk in, put his fingers inside me, make me come and walk out again, leaving me there with my red bum in the air. White, naked and vulnerable but always sage.

Conrad's dick grew again.

I put it in my mouth and sucked him, smiling with my eyes.

He fucked me again.

'I knew you were a bad girl.'

'Nonsense. I'm just your run-of-the-mill pro-porn feminist with transgressive leanings and an eye on the future of the revolution.'

'You are?'

'Oh yes. I don't think it is possible for women to be genuinely progressive unless they have accepted the truth of their sexuality, placed it in the public domain and then built the agenda from that truth. That is, if the thinkers who construct these ideas cannot make themselves sophisticated with the knowledge of sexual truth, then they cannot impact reality. Furthermore, feminists seek to remove the pleasure out of everything and I see it as my personal mission to bring it back.'

'Rather difficult being a masochist and a feminist,' he observed.

'I don't feel that I am a masochist in any psychically dangerous way,' I answered. 'I feel that I am mastering my own truth and there is nothing to be ashamed of. And I think this is particularly important in the light of a political climate made reactionary by AIDS.'

'Well,' he said with a smile, 'you are a one.'

When we went downstairs, everybody had gone. Aunt Susan was inspecting cigarette burns and Mrs Erin was sweeping up broken glass. It had turned into quite a party. Granny would have been very gratified. She loved funerals.

Conrad and I kissed in the hallway.

'I will ring you in London,' he said.

I watched him drive his dreadful Morris Minor down the drive.

'Is that the one who writes for the papers?' Aunt Susan said.

Granny left me her Austin Healey so now I had a cool car, a furious dog, some deco jet jewellery, a bizarre fur coat, a box camera and several vintage designer hats which the Aunt Susan said were 'worth a fortune'.

Now I am her, I said, as I drove the car to London, well over the speed limit, as she always had, and with a cocktail shaker on my knee, as she had, and Owen in the passenger seat with his head out of the window, tongue flapping, ears pushed back by the wind.

10. 1987–8

Crowds of people had arrived with half truths and unpleasant truths. An inadequate hero and an unknowable mother. They had both died in misery. I was haunted. January came and everything was grey. The skies pressed down; there was only cold and rain and the dark, and the days were all as one.

It was as if messages were arriving from deep within my body; they were not borne of cold intellect or even identifiable memories, but they arrived from some unknowable place, pushing forward, inchoate and unreadable, but able to be pushed down again, firmly, with a harsh intake of cigarette smoke, or a vodka, or Granny's drugs. I worked through these inordinate pharmaceuticals with reckless abandon. Sometimes they made me violently sick, but they rarely let me down. I was mad and wild and completely liberated.

Sometimes I woke up at three o'clock and thought it was after lunch; sometimes I lost a day, sometimes I wondered why it was always so dark, had there been some kind of an apocalyptic episode while I had been unconscious?

I only watched one video and that was *The Rocky Horror Picture Show*. It played on a permanent loop. I gazed at the freaks and knew they were right. I saw deep and mystical meaning in the screenplay, the ultimate manifesto for sexual individualism all wrapped up in the subtext of subversion written by a genius. I sang the songs to myself and knew I would have been happy in that castle with Frank and the others. I would have liked to have been whipped by that weird butler. I would have made a great Nell. God knows you didn't have to sing very well; just cavort about with make-up on and suspenders showing and I pretty much did that as a lifestyle choice.

If I went out it was to walk with Owen and/or pull men out of bars. They appear in my diaries as names only and some of them are difficult to recall but I guess they were the kind who didn't mind a mad woman as long as they could fuck her. I was a free prostitute and I am sure they were glad of it, but I never found out anything about them.

The episodes were a welcome distraction from the isolation and morbidity. The men didn't mind that the flat was junkie untidy. They weren't looking for a lifetime bond, they were looking for a slut fuck.

I didn't think about love at this time; I wasn't aware of wanting affection. I didn't actually want anyone close, I wanted them to keep their distance but fuck me all the same. It was all about the mechanics of release and the relief of distraction.

There was a David and a Dan and a Miles and a Joe. I remember doing it on the floor with one of them. Stocky bloke with biceps and a shaved head. He liked German noise bands and was quite hardcore in his tastes. Not my type usually. I like thin and dark and effete and bisexual – a kind of cross between a liquorice stick and a drag queen. He was more pint down the pub, roll up and two years in the army. He taught philosophy so he wasn't thick. I didn't have to lower my game. Lowering one's game is always a sexual turn off. I find that now, even now I am old. I have never been attracted to the thick youth with muscle and erection. I would rather have less sex and more travel. I can surrender nightly orgasm as long as there are exchanges of new ideas. Middle-aged men don't always feel the same, of course. They don't want to chat, they want to fuck. Now they can thanks to Pfizer.

This stocky bloke pinned my arms behind my head and I wrapped my legs around his waist and we fucked on the floor in the kitchen, then again on the kitchen table. Him, whoever he was, behind. And me with my face pressed down on the painted wood. I grabbed onto the edges of the table with my hands. The pepper mill crashed onto the floor.

I spread my legs good and wide, opened myself up, so he could have taken me anywhere. He was traditional. He grabbed my labia, pushed his palm against my clitoris and rubbed it with unbearable determination so that all thought of escape left, and I had to dance with him because he had the control. He rubbed me and, as I started to lose it, he pushed his penis into me. He had a wide white arse, wide pelvis and a strong push. He knew what he was doing, was co-ordinated and, as he pushed the delicious hard head into me, he rubbed me, tuned in and forced us to mutual climax.

He wanted to see me again actually, and I complied because he was a spectacular fuck, and they don't come along that often, despite what you read in fiction. Neither is it something you can assess from either personality or appearance. I've seen the most useless-looking individual become more than useful when divested. And the other way around. There are many who think they are a lot better in bed than they are, enabled to be so by polite women.

Once *he*, can't remember the name, came to my house when I had pornography on the video. Porn was becoming quite cool in the late 80s. It was seen as a conduit through which to ask questions, it was connected to interesting technology and relevant civil-rights arguments. Larry Flynt was a hip anti-hero. I watched quite a lot of it, mostly gay, thanks to the fact that it belonged to Kevin the hairdresser. I also bought spanking films from Janus in Soho.

I liked the way they checked out my arse in there and sometimes went in purely to bend over and show them my cheeks. I wished one of them would have grabbed me and taken a hairbrush to my flesh, but that is not the protocol of the porn parlour, unfortunately. They have to have some boundaries in real life at least.

I was pure and white and slightly frustrated. As I had not seen Daddy for months, I had not been taken in hand. So I watched spanking vids, where the girls were great but the men were combed over and in upsetting trousers and would have put me off the whole pastime completely if it hadn't been hardwired into my brain.

He, can't remember the name, became politically correct annoyed, saying that porn was not subversive, whatever the aging punks may think, but merely served to reinforce a status quo where women were empty holes.

'Pornography,' I said, 'exists because society cannot accept its sexuality. It is cultivated by repression and denial. If the secret complexities of needs and desires were accepted and celebrated, there would be no need to provide this means of crude education and haphazard arousal. Look to pre-communist China if you wish to see how the erotic arts should be displayed – without shame and as a means of attaining virtues such as temperance and generosity. Porn,' I went on, 'has only existed since erotica was banned, in 1857 to be exact, with the Obscene Publications Act. Porn is not porn's problem, it is your problem. If you weren't so scared and uptight and confused you would know that.'

He, can't remember the name, accused me of being stupid, as men do when they can't think of an answer. Then he started complaining that I only wanted him for the sex and I said what was wrong with that? He said he wanted more than that. He wanted a relationship. I said I did not know what he was talking about. I didn't know what a relationship was, beyond a word to describe the fact that two people were interacting on some level. Relationship surely was a subjective issue whose description was subject to the reality of the individual, like beauty or evil. He was the philosopher, surely he could see the meaninglessness of 'relationship' as a descriptive word.

He told me I was out of touch with myself and left.

He was replaced by other faces and dicks and the latter were easier to remember. I had no time for the small ones, I'm afraid. I just didn't. Not time, no patience, no tolerance. I was such a bitch. No wonder I needed to be punished.

I learned to tolerate the medium sizes, achieve some semblance of politeness. But it was the big ones for which I was always genuinely grateful. The big dicks got my full attention; sometimes they received an emotion akin to love. What a lovely surprise it was when one unwrapped the package to find one's mouth crammed with hard meat. They choked me and they poked me.

The irony is, of course, that it was these men who did not need encouragement or gratitude; it was their less lucky brothers with the smaller endowments who required the love of a good woman. I was not a good woman and neither did I have any aspirations to be so. I had no aspirations. My expectations were low and they had been largely met.

I remember the sensations of hard shaft inside me, grinding and pumping, and sometimes letting myself go into them. I do not remember the nature of the orgasm. Orgasms are difficult to recall, their essence seems to require the present. One has to be there and then they go. I have a lot of different kinds of orgasm, which men never believe, possibly because they only have one kind. I can certainly have an orgasm that is a purely emotional release, the physical sensation being only a part of it. I can have an internal orgasm by mistake when the top of a dick presses against some nerve ending deep inside and lets me go. And then there are the mechanics of the clitoral, always reliable and completely controllable. The goodnight self-fuck. The vibe to fantasy. The sheer bliss of self-release, so satisfying in the knowledge that one is so self-contained. Self-release sometimes made me long for Daddy's dick but it also confirmed the fact that I no longer needed him. As far as I was concerned, he had abandoned me when I needed him and failed me in ways that were too painful to assess let alone describe to anyone.

I cannot remember who gave me which kind of orgasm, but I know that the releases I had with Daddy were the best and most varied and the nearest to meaningful love. Daddy allowed me to be me, and I allowed him to look.

I was wearing shorts at this time, little black satin shorts, long socks, high boots and tailored jackets with collared shirts. It was a good look and I always had a school tie, which often came in useful when I was out with Kevin. My hair had sprouted out of the neat Louise Brooks bob that Daddy had designed into a boyish short back and sides with a long fringe thanks to Kevin the hairdresser who had taken control. He discouraged me from promiscuous pursuits. His best friend had died of AIDS and he told me that the disease had killed everybody in New York.

'You were monogamous when you were fucking Daddy,' he commented. 'And happier! Though your hair wasn't as good.'

I stared into the mirror. I was wearing a pair of Ray-Bans and sitting behind a cloud of smoke so it was difficult to see my face. Frankie Goes to Hollywood was on quite loud.

'You're a slut,' he said. 'I respect that, but it's dangerous out there, trust me.'

I had a test and was clear and carried on fucking.

Dan liked to bite my thighs and ejaculate into my arsehole. Simon did it doggie.

Lorne wrote poetry and had a filthy mouth. He was one of the few men who could make me come on the telephone. Telephone sex was his favourite. He lived in Brent so it was easier for him, I suppose. Saved the effort and expense of travel.

'How's my filthy tart?'

'She has her fingers down her panties.'

'I should come round there and give you a good fucking. Would you like that, would you like to suck my hard cock?'

'I want your hard cock. I want you to fuck me and come all over me. I have my hands round it now.'

'Are your fingers in your panties?'

'Yes.'

'Put them in yourself. I want to hear you come.'

And so on. Sometimes he said poetry to me, which I found more embarrassing than giving him head on a park bench. It was like stand-up comedy without the jokes. I didn't know where to put myself.

I also had 'relations' with a hairy biker, which was Kevin's fault being as I met him with Kevin in a basement club in Hackney. It was all very well Kevin the hairdresser lecturing me about sleazy sex, but he was never out of low-down places himself. The biker was a leather-clad heterosexual top. What more could one ask for?

I bent over the seat of his Norton and gave him my ass. Luckily for him I was wearing a leather miniskirt, stockings, suspenders, stilettos and no pants. He had access and he took it, pulling his hard-on out of his leathers and giving it to me. The bike shuddered and clattered. It was going to fall over, so he pushed me over a fire escape. Me on the steps, buttocks up, him in me, grabbing my waist. Giving me a good hard informal seeing to. I saw him again.

He made me go to this council flat in Hackney and serve him beers on a tray in front of his biker friends. I don't think they were bikers in the *Easy Rider* sense of the word. I think they were losers who happened to own third-hand motorbikes. One of them had a mother in Parson's Green. I don't think they were outlaws. Mechanics probably, if I had to guess.

Still, they were rude enough to get an atmosphere going. I had to slave it up for my alpha friend, wear a little grey skirt and a pinny and high black patent walking shoes with stripy socks. My pants, white and cotton, were wet. He really excited me. He was so crude and unpredictable; there was a genuine danger that I had not sensed for some time, not since I had first met Daddy and I did not know who he was or how far he would go. The biker ripped my shirt open with one meat hand so the buttons flew off and my tits were everywhere. I remained unflustered, merely staring at him with an expression somewhere between contempt and ennui, which drove him crazy. He put his mouth round my nipples and sucked, his friends all looking on, gaping, gawping and gratified. My legs buckled slightly. I don't think they could quite believe it. I certainly couldn't.

They all looked suitably impressed and more so when he sent me to his bedroom, left the door open, followed me in and fucked me so that they could hear it happening. A couple of slaps, a lot of begging. We were quite loud.

'Do you want more?' he enquired.

'Why not?' I replied.

He sent the others in, one by one. I was on my stomach, so I didn't look at them, and didn't want to. It wasn't their faces I was after, and I certainly didn't want to kiss them. But I did like their hard dicks in me; I liked the fact that they arrived excited and desperate for me. Well, not me, let's be clear – my shameless orifice, which had been well pumped up by their friend and was now being offered.

They were mostly quite ugly, but they were hard and rough and strong, so being taken from the back by this over-excited trio was very gratifying. I had never experienced a rogering quite like it, though, having discovered it, I have been to orgies since and instigated the same type of drama. I did make them wear condoms. I had listened to Kevin.

There was a lot of juice, which is not my favourite thing, and I had to have a bath in the biker's flat. He had a pink plastic bath and there was a scum of limescale around the taps. The shower, if that is what it was, was clogged up and produced only a dribble. There are limits. The bathroom put me off in the end, that and his beard. We didn't achieve formal closure, but simply stopped making dates. Nobody minded. Though I couldn't hazard a guess at the nature of his internal life. I dread to think. He behaved like a pig so he probably was one. I told Kevin all about it and he said he had had one or two of them as well. He agreed with me about the bathroom. There are limits.

So, one father dead, Daddy lover nowhere to be seen and Granny buried in the garden, I took the barbiturates and slept with everybody. But then the grief started to arrive in waves.

The telephone rang and rang and I left it.

I did what one does. Cried, lay down, hugged Owen, cried, lay down, watched television, starved, slept, drank, stopped going out and putting it about.

I took Granny's pills like Dr Jekyll experimenting with myself to see how far I could go.

Then Daddy rang.

'Who? My daddy's dead. Frank Black is an ex parrot,' I slurred.

'Stella, listen to me, I am coming round in twenty minutes and if you don't open the door I'm ringing the police.'

'But you're dead.'

Jimmy picked the lock.

Daddy found me face down on the sofa with Owen whining beside me.

He physically lifted me up and put me in the car. Jimmy drove us back to Cheyne Walk.

I was tucked up and given Lucozade, a comic and a good talking to.

A doctor came. My blood pressure was taken and said to be dangerously low. I thought I had been fainting because of the drugs. Apparently not. Decisions were made but I paid no attention. I slept.

Now I was the ill one.

Different illness, of course, being mental.

I cried a lot. Daddy made me eat. He let me smoke but not in the bedroom so I had to go to the drawing room in my nightie. I lay on the sofa, underneath a tartan blanket, with Owen who liked Daddy. I would be in a foetal position, with my thumb in my mouth and my head on his lap.

Daddy was firm and gentle. He threw away all Granny's pills, delivering a lecture as he did so, but I still had no reality. Sometimes I was his little girl and he looked after me. Sometimes I was a grown-up making plans.

He allowed me the full range of self-pity, which should be allowed. I was alone after all. I had nobody.

'Where were you?' I accused. 'You just went and then you never came back.'

'Stella, that isn't fair. I went to Hong Kong as I told you I had to. I rang you the day I came back. I continued to ring you but there was either no answer or the phone was off the hook.'

'You could have written, or come round.'

'I did come round, actually, more than once. Then I saw a man coming out of the house and I wasn't going to submit myself to your whims and rejection. I assumed you had moved on. I had no idea you were miserable.'

'Did you miss me?'

'Of course I missed you. I love you. Plus I was very worried. Something wasn't right.'

I told him about Granny's funeral and the debts and Owen and Aunt Susan. He thought it was all exasperating. He was cross about the mismanagement of the family money even though I said I didn't mind.

'You're young, Stella,' he said. 'You don't understand.'

Not that young any more. Getting older all the time. The stress was beginning to show in my face. Things were happening to my neck that reminded me of Wes Craven movies.

'Do stop looking at yourself in the mirror,' he would admonish. 'You're not some dippy fashion model.'

It took me a year to recover. By the time of my twenty-ninth birthday I was less dishevelled, less scared, more able to cope. I could go out. I could walk around with Daddy and Owen. Daddy had become obsessed with Owen, which I took as a sign of his aging. He always needed to know where I was and where Owen was at every point in the day. He went to Harrods and bought Owen a range of designer accessories and expensive china bowls with bone motif. Before I knew it there was a dog walker and a speciality grooming salon. Owen was approaching middle age and had mellowed.

The sex was different too, not with Owen obviously, with Daddy. There were no games now. I hadn't the creative energy or the libido. Daddy did fuck me, but slow and gentle, using his dick to make me come rather than his mind to turn me on. There were no more slaps or punishment play although he did tell me off a lot and make decisions for me, which I enjoyed.

He made me go to bed early and have early suppers and told me exactly what to eat. There were suppers on trays and healthy portions. If I complained, he threatened me but he never followed through.

We played it straight: vanilla, no hanky-panky-spanky. He retained his authority and instructed me sternly about eating and sleeping. I was an invalid. He still had the control. I liked it like that and so did he.

I started to emerge in the spring of 1989. Details became illuminated and I could look at them without feeling fear. I saw beauty and I also saw that Daddy looked older. Grey hair, thinning shoulders, stooped, liver spots, occasionally forgetting things I had told him only the day before. We started to repeat conversations. He became fussier and more fastidious and more concerned about his possessions. If we had to go anywhere there were endless conversations about routes. He spent his time telling me what was in the *Daily Telegraph* or discussing how best to clean his decanters. He fussed about candle wax and the positions of chairs and how you couldn't get a decent shirt any more. I became more bored. I did not want to be his little girl any more. I wanted to go back to America.

'Big mistake,' he told me. 'You are vulnerable. You've been very ill. Believe me, Stella, I've seen breakdowns. Not everybody gets their life back. You have to be careful. Dr Meadows says.'

Daddy wanted to hold onto his vulnerable little girl. On some level he did not want me to grow up. We still adored each other but there had been a shift. The kink occasionally came back; certainly he remained dominant, certainly I enjoyed having to do what I was told because it made me feel protected, certainly we still turned each other on. But we were both more fragile and more careful. He had been wounded by Mandy; I had been wounded by life and death. He still held me close and he was always the man in bed, but we did not play as we once had.

By June I was well and I wanted to go forward. I loved him but the energy was pushing me away from him. I couldn't see a future with him. Well, I could, but that was the problem: I could see a future with him. I could see it and it comprised of being with him in one of two houses, talking to his friends and knowing all the details of my destiny. It would have been comfortable but it would not have been an adventure.

I wasn't a trophy wife; I wasn't a hostess; I wasn't a mother. We would have had no projects to share, no mutual interests and no common reference points. I couldn't overcome these facts.

'Conrad will pay me to help with his new book,' I said. 'It's reading, it's not even a job. He will pay me enough. It will only be six months. Six months in libraries.'

'I don't even know Conrad,' Daddy said. 'Is he safe?'

About as safe as gelignite, I thought, but did not say so. His last book had caused two policemen to be imprisoned. Now he was investigating the IRA's finances. He had received a large advance and several death threats.

'You won't come back,' said Daddy. 'You will go to America and you won't come back.'

I knew this was true.

I knew that Kevin the hairdresser's friend Colin wanted to rent my flat.

I knew that Conrad fancied me.

I wanted to go.

Daddy and I were not going to grow old together, I knew that. The smells were wrong. The timing was wrong. The age difference was wrong.

I smoked five cigarettes while I was telling him. We were at his house in the country.

He looked out of the window onto the rolling green of his land and I sensed that he was perceiving loneliness.

He turned back towards me and to my horror I saw tears running down his face. I didn't know what to do. I was appalled and I felt sick. My head swam as, disorientated, I watched as I might have watched an unfamiliar mammal appear in the jungle. I froze, wondering what was going to happen next.

He didn't sob, thank God, but he looked heartbroken. I knew he loved me, as I loved him. But because I was now departing, I had assumed he would be as easy with the idea as I was.

I couldn't stay with a future full of disease and decrepitude and the gothic possibilities of immobility. I wasn't someone who foresaw nursing, unless there were Benny Hill overtones and experimentation with lewd procedure and weird equipment.

'I am middle aged,' he observed, 'not geriatric. But you are right. This fantasy must end and you must go or risk being suffocated. I love you too much to hurt you. And, ironically, I am too old for you. You will never settle down, Stella. And I don't think that matters as long as you're happy. You will always be beautiful because, even when you are older, you will have personality and panache.'

'And fantastic tits,' I said.

'And fantastic tits,' he agreed.

*   *   *

Conrad met me at the airport. He was wearing a mac.

'It rains in Washington,' he said.

Great, I thought, I've got all the wrong shoes.

'Is that all your luggage? Christ, you always were a gypsy.'

I had one small overnight case.

'I can buy things when I'm there,' I said.

'Not on what I'm paying you.'

He smiled and hugged me. 'I'm glad you're here.'

He had the tickets. 'Give me your passport,' he said, 'and do your buttons up. I can see your bra.'

'I don't wear a bra.'

He bent down and looked closely. 'Oh no, my mistake, well, you should and don't answer back.'

I pouted, but did as I was told while he continued to stare possessively at my breasts.

'And don't sulk.'

He gave me money for sweets and we flew first class.